Inverse Abdominoplasty

Kemal Tunc Tiryaki
Editor

Inverse Abdominoplasty

An Illustrated Guide

Springer

Editor
Kemal Tunc Tiryaki
Department of Plastic Surgery
Cellest Plastic Surgery Center
Istanbul
Turkey

ISBN 978-3-319-39308-7 ISBN 978-3-319-39310-0 (eBook)
DOI 10.1007/978-3-319-39310-0

Library of Congress Control Number: 2016956706

Printed on acid-free paper

This Springer imprint is published by Springer Nature
The registered company is Springer International Publishing AG Switzerland
The registered company address is: Gewerbestrasse 11, 6330 Cham, Switzerland

Acknowledgments

I was contemplating about penning together a book that would define abdominal beauty and what it takes to surgically recreate it for some time, but it was only when an offer came from Springer Verlag that I seriously considered doing it. Theirs was a perfect timing, right after the American-Brazilian Meeting in 2015, where I had a presentation on abdominal beauty and the surgical maneuvers to fashion the abdominal shape and shadows, which we finally find beautiful.

All throughout this time, I took a great pleasure working on this book, and I am particularly proud of putting together such a great team of authors for this project.

I owe a great deal of what I know to my experience from my fellowship with Dr. Osman Oymak, with whom I am working together since 1999. It is Osman, who patiently taught me aesthetic plastic surgery operations, as well as many other details like the art of patient relationships and care.

However I would never have had the chance to work together with him had not I been in the masterful guiding hands of my professor of residency, Dr. Adnan Uzunismail. Under his supervision I became the plastic reconstructive surgeon, who could put this book together with my fellow authors.

I want to thank also Dr. Nazım Cerkes and Dr. Renato Saltz for their inspiration for me to try to teach and share everything I do and I learn. Last but not least, I thank my wife Sylvia and my son Teodor for their continuous support.

Foreword

It is an honor and great privilege to write this foreword. Dr. Tunc Tiryaki is a renowned educator, forward thinker, and internationally recognized leader in aesthetic plastic surgery.

I have known Tunc for many years and have always been very impressed with his surgical skills; outstanding teaching abilities; and his creative, innovative mind. He has distinguished himself not only in his native city of Istanbul but throughout the world.

Obesity, childbearing, and sedentary life can affect the abdominal muscles, abdominal fat, and skin in many different negative ways. Abdominoplasty combined with liposuction and other body contouring techniques is an effective, safe way to restore the original "core anatomy," to improve torso contouring, and to provide long-term good functional and cosmetic improvements never achievable by diet and exercise only. These patients are so happy and motivated with their "new appearance," and they become addicted to healthier diets, exercise, and a completely healthier life – these are some of the happiest patients I have in my practice! In the morbid obese group of patients, studies have shown a significant long-term loss of weight, spontaneous recovery from many illnesses like diabetes and hypertension, improvement in cardiovascular risk factors, and a reduction in mortality.

Plastic and reconstructive surgeons have risen to the occasion and have developed new and safe techniques to help this group of patients dealing with poor muscle anatomy and redundant skin and fat on their abdomens. Similar to what we have witnessed in the past when innovative techniques in craniofacial, microsurgery, and endoscopic surgery have emerged to face reconstructive and cosmetic challenges in burns, cancer, and trauma.

Dr. Tiryaki has assembled a group of knowledgeable experts who have contributed to this comprehensive and practical text covering all aspects of modern and safe abdominoplasty. Of particular interest is the fact he has included young colleagues among renowned experienced authors who have published extensively in this challenging topic.

His text has many interesting chapters. I call your attention for the first few dealing with the functional and surgical anatomy, the chapters on interesting new concepts of forces and tension to create beauty, and many new options and techniques in abdominoplasty. The final chapters deal with the combination of procedures, prevention of complications, and the critical postoperative care to avoid infection, hematomas, and the always feared deep venous thrombosis and pulmonary embolism.

Congratulations to Dr. Tunc Tiryaki and the very distinguished group of authors for this landmark contribution to aesthetic plastic surgery. This is a must-have book to all the novice and also the experienced cosmetic surgeons that specialize in body contouring surgery.

Salt Lake City, Utah Renato Saltz

Contents

Chapter 1
Surgical Anatomy of the Abdominal Wall

Derya Bingöl, Ozay Ozkaya Mutlu, and Osman Oymak

The objective of this chapter is to concentrate the attention of the reader on particular anatomical details of the abdominal wall, which are important for the surgical perspective.

As such, the abdomen constitutes the part of the body between the thorax and pelvis. The outline of the anterior abdominal wall is approximately hexagonal in shape. It is bounded superiorly by the arched costal margin, laterally by the midaxillary lines on either side bilaterally, and the anterior abdominal wall is in continuity, by the anterior half of the iliac crest, inguinal ligament, pubic crest, and pubic symphysis, inferiorly [1].

Externally, there are three basic anatomical landmarks in the abdominal area. These lines are demarking the grooves and eminences of the abdominal area. In order to mimic this ideal anatomy and to create a beautiful result, these structures are to be recreated (Fig. 1.1).

1.1 Linea Semilunaris

The linea semilunares can be seen as a pair of linear impressions in the skin that correspond with the lateral most edges of the rectus abdominis. It is formed by the

D. Bingöl, MD
Plastic, Reconstructive and Aesthetic Surgery Clinic, Medikal Park Hospital, Bursa, Turkey

O.O. Mutlu, MD
Plastic, Reconstructive and Aesthetic Surgery Clinic, Okmeydanı Training and Research Hospital, Istanbul, Turkey

O. Oymak (✉)
Oymak Plastic Surgery Clinic (OPC), Istanbul, Turkey
e-mail: osmanoymak@opc.com.tr

K.T. Tiryaki (ed.), *Inverse Abdominoplasty*, DOI 10.1007/978-3-319-39310-0_1

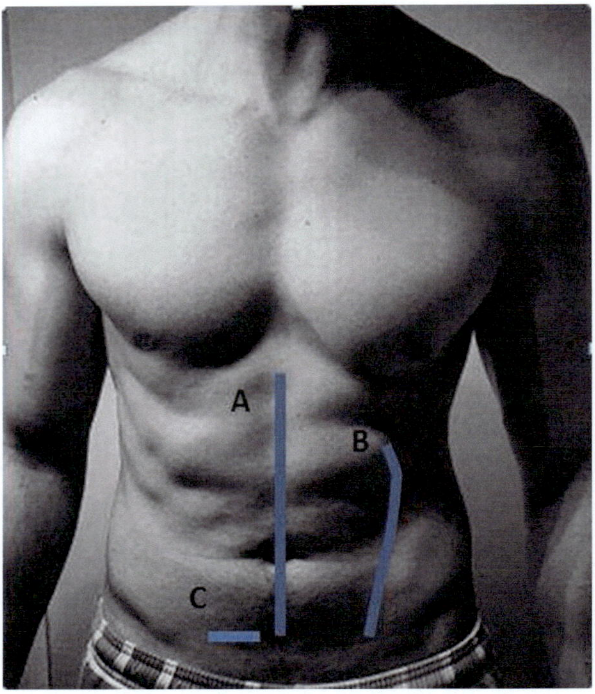

Fig. 1.1 *A* Linea alba *B* Linea semilunaris *C* Arcuate line

band of aponeuroses of the external oblique, the internal oblique, and transverse abdominal muscles [2].

1.2 Arcuate Line

The arcuate line is defined by the most inferior extension of the posterior rectus sheath, forming a crescent-shaped border. The arcuate line is generally located two fingerbreadths from the umbilicus to midway between the umbilicus and pubis. There are reports in the literature, however, that state the arcuate line is closer to 75 % of the distance between pubic crest to umbilicus or 1.8 cm superior to the anterior superior iliac spine [3]. It is not visible from the exterior [3].

1.3 Linea Alba

In the midline, a slight furrow extends from the xiphoid process above, to the pubic symphysis below, representing the linea alba in the abdominal wall. The fibres of the anterior and posterior sheaths of the rectus muscle interlace at the midline, forming the linea alba.

From the surgical anatomical perspective, the abdominal wall consists of various structural layers.

1.4 Layers of the Abdominal Wall

From the surgical anatomical perspective, the abdominal wall consists of various layers, namely, the skin, superficial fascia, fat, muscles, the transversalis fascia, and the parietal peritoneum.

1.4.1 Skin and Subcutaneous Tissue

This outmost layer consists of the skin, superficial fat layer, the fascia superficialis (Scarpa's fascia), and the deep fat layer.

1.4.1.1 Skin

Epidermis The epidermis is formed of five layers, and the epithelial cells transform itself into a keratin layer, which constantly peels off.

Dermis The deeper structure called the dermis has two layers with no threshold between them. They are:

- The *papillary* layer which is thinner and external
- The *reticular* layer which is deeper and denser

The skin covering the anterior abdominal wall is thin, in comparison with that of the back, and is relatively mobile over the underlying structural layers except at the umbilical region, where it is fixed. The thickness of the abdominal skin seems to augment when approaching the midline and especially around the umbilicus. Natural elastic traction lines of the skin (also known as skin tension lines or Kraissl's lines) of the anterior abdominal wall are disposed transversely. Above the level of the umbilicus, these tension lines extend mostly in a horizontal direction, while below this level, they continue along with a slight inferomedial oblique direction. Incisions made along, or parallel to, these lines tend to heal without much scarring, whereas incisions that cross these lines tend to result in wide or heaped-up scars [1].

1.4.1.2 Superficial Fat Layer (Superficial Adipose Tissue)

Superficial fat, just under the dermis, is formed of large fat lobes encased between fibrous septa in a honeycomb-like structure and presents nearly constant characteristics throughout. These septa (retinacula cutis superficialis or Camper`s fascia)

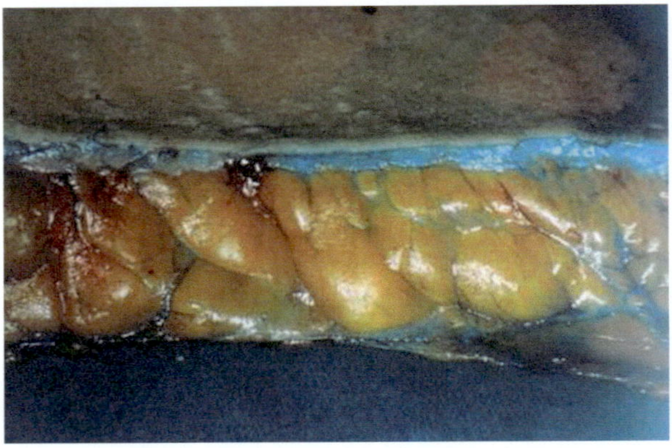

Fig. 1.2 Retinacula cutis superficialis or Camper's fascia

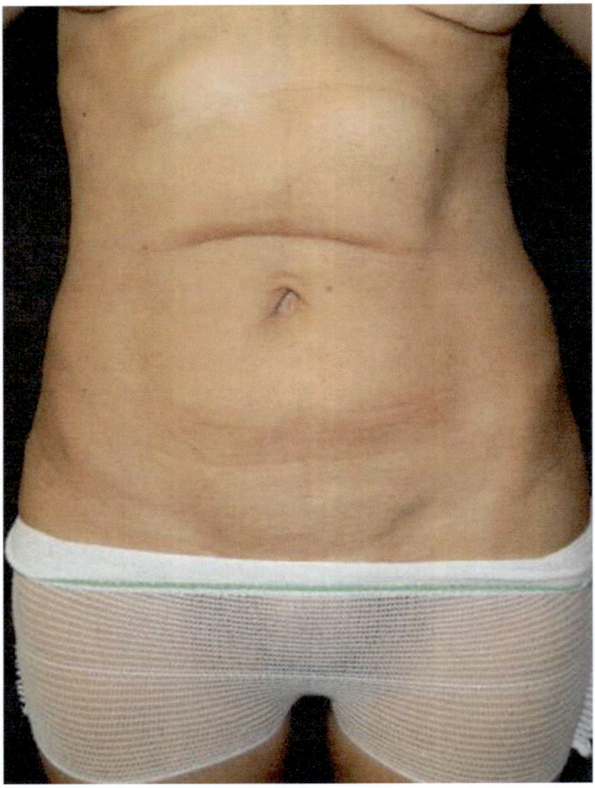

Fig. 1.3 The attachments of Camper's fascia to the skin above the umbilicus can occasionally create a deep horizontal line

appear well defined. They are mostly oriented perpendicular to the surface and are mechanically strong, anchoring the dermis to the deeper planes (Fig. 1.2).

Stronger attachments to the dermis in the midline and above the umbilicus have been reported [4]. This is the reason why liposuction performed above the umbilicus and close to the midline is more prone to result in irregularities. The attachments of the retinacula cutis superficialis to the skin at 5–7 cm above the umbilicus can occasionally be stronger than usual and create a deep horizontal line. This deformity cannot be corrected by classical or scarpa-saving undermining – more superficial interventions are necessary (Fig. 1.3).

Things to Remember
- In order to mimic this ideal anatomy and to create a beautiful result, the superficial landmarks are to be recreated.
- Liposuction performed above the umbilicus and close to the midline is more prone to irregularities.
- On rare occasions particularly above the umbilicus, the retinacula cutis superficialis' attachments to the skin may be stronger than usual and create a deep horizontal line.
- This deformity cannot be corrected by classical or scarpa-saving undermining – more superficial interventions are necessary.

1.4.1.3 Fascia Superficialis (Scarpa's Fascia)

The superficial fascia comprises two distinct layers: an outer, adipose layer lying subjacent to the dermis and an inner fibroelastic layer termed Scarpa's fascia, the membranous layer of superficial fascia [1]. The fibrous layer with a membranous appearance –the fascia superficialis – is continuous and well organized. It separates the superficial and deep adipose tissues (Fig. 1.4).

This layer can be followed as a dissection plane from the thorax to the inguinal ligament. It does not appear uniform in thickness. Being a well-defined white layer in the lower abdomen, thickening toward the inguinal ligament where a multilayered structure of multidirectional collagen bundles is perceptible. The Scarpa's fascia loses consistency in the upper abdomen, where it can be identified as a much thinner translucid collagen layer through which adipose tissue can be seen [4]. This membrane, which is strongly fused medially to the linea alba and caudally to the

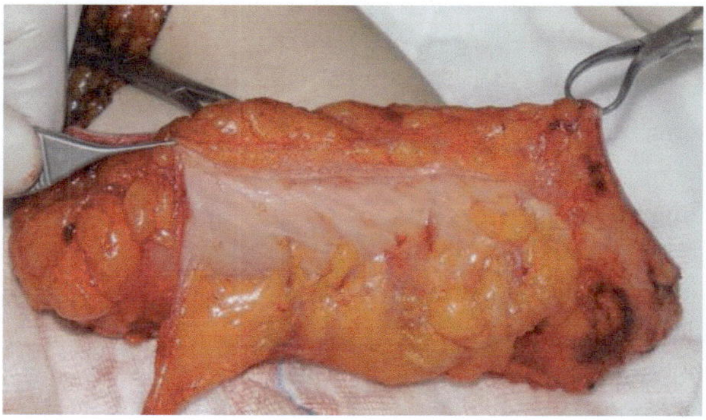

Fig. 1.4 Scarpa's fascia

inguinal ligament and the osseous prominence of the iliac crest, cranially continues into the thorax. The membranous layer (Scarpa's fascia) is an important structure, which is strong enough to diminish the tension of sutures when identified and sutured in continuity during closure of the abdominal flap [5].

1.4.1.4 Deep Fat Layer (Deep Adipose Tissue, DAT)

Deep adipose tissue appears very different from the superficial adipose tissue, as its fat lobes are smaller, flatter, and less well defined (Fig. 1.5). This adipose layer shows significant variations in terms of thickness between different areas. Towards the points, at which the membranous layer of the subcutaneous tissue adheres to salient structures (e.g., the inguinal ligament, bony prominences, linea alba), they become thinner and tend to progressively reduce the fat component. However, the network of collagen fibres (retinacula cutis profunda) become stronger and more tightly packed and connects the deep aspect of the membranous layer to the deep fascia.

In the deep adipose layer, the fibrous septa are predominantly obliquely and horizontally oriented (retinacula cutis profunda) and connect the membranous layer (Scarpa's fascia) to the fascia of the rectus abdominis or external oblique muscle [4]. The membranous layers DAT and SAT create a sliding system that absorb the mechanical stimulations applied to the skin or that are generated by muscular contractions.

In this way the subcutaneous tissue ensures autonomy between the skin and the muscles. If any scarring creates adhesion between the skin, membranous layer, and deep fascia, every muscular contraction could also affect the skin, activating the cutaneous receptors – also vice versa: every stimulation of the skin could be transmitted to the underlying structures. This may explain the importance of the correct layered reconstruction of the subcutaneous tissue in avoiding complications after closure of the abdominal surgery wounds [4].

Things to Remember

1. A trilaminar structure is always present at the abdominal subcutis.
2. Over the rectus abdominis muscle, there is a thicker region, and the difference is mainly attributable to the superficial compartment.
3. The deep fat compartment has a minor contribution to the overall thickness, which is less than 25 % of the total thickness.
4. The superficial fat compartment is more susceptible to increase in thickness in obesity compared with the deep compartment.
5. The Scarpa's fascia is always present and does not become vestigial with increased adiposity [6].

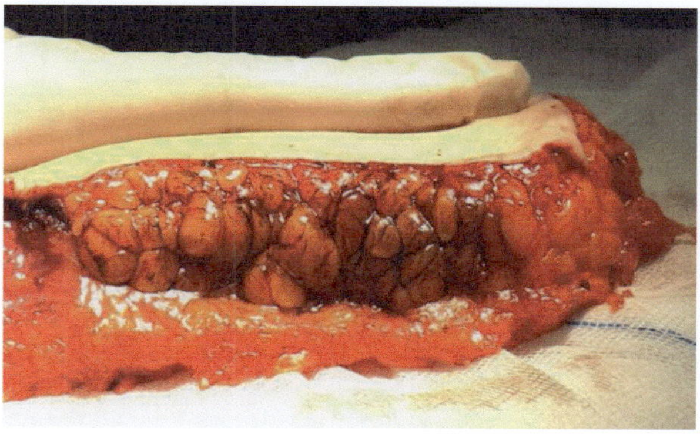

Fig. 1.5 Deep adipose tissue appears very different from the superficial adipose tissue, as its fat lobes are smaller, flatter, and less well defined

1.5 Musculofascial System of the Abdomen

The abdominal wall consists of five paired muscles: three flat muscles and two vertical muscles. The three flat muscles are the external oblique, internal oblique, and the transversus abdominis. The two vertical muscles are the rectus abdominis and pyramidalis. The three-layered structure, combined with extensive aponeuroses, works in a synkinetic fashion. Fusion of the fascial layers of these muscles forms three distinct fascial lines: the linea alba and two semilunar lines. The linea alba is formed by the fusion of both rectus sheaths at the midline, while the semilunar lines are formed by the union of the internal oblique, transversus abdominis, and external oblique as they join the rectus sheath (Fig. 1.6).

The abdominal muscular anatomy is well known with one vertical muscle anteriorly and three large lateral muscles overlying each other inversely. The vertical rectus muscle is divided by the linea alba.

1.5.1 Linea Alba

The linea alba is the rest of the embryonic ventral suture made up of three distinct aponeurotic layers originating from three lateral abdominal muscles, migrating to the midline, encircling the rectus abdominis muscle and fusing in the midline. It is a three-dimensional composition of tendon fibres from abdominal wall muscles. The cranial aspect is attached to the xiphoid process of the sternum, while caudally, it inserts at the pubic symphysis. This strong attachment to the sternum prevents any hyperextension of the vertebral structures. Also, the midline insertions of these fibres play a significant role in stabilizing the abdominal wall [2, 7].

According to the orientation of the collagen fibres, the linea alba is organized into three laminae: the anterior, the middle, and the posterior laminas. Substantial amounts of elastic fibres are in all the laminae at all levels of the linea alba. The elastic fibres

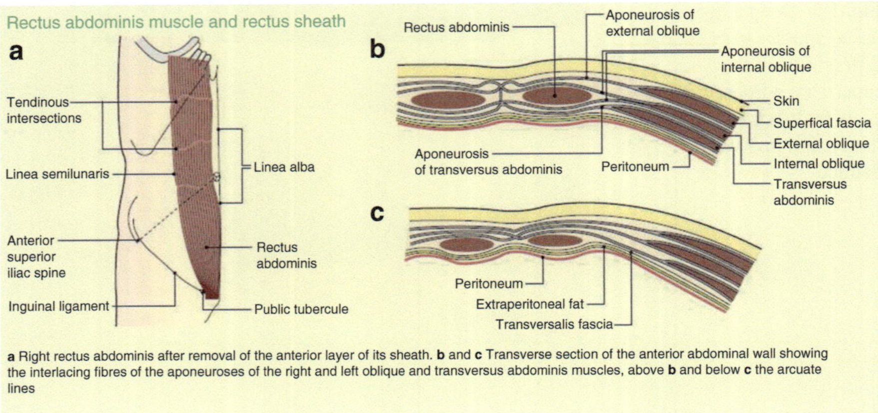

Fig. 1.6 Musculofascial system of the abdomen. (**a**) Right rectus abdominis after removal of the anterior layer of its sheath. (**b**, **c**) Transverse sections of the anterior abdominal wall showing the interlacing fibres of the aponeuroses of the right and left oblique and transversus abdominis muscles, above (**b**) and below (**c**) the arcuate lines (Source: Moore [19])

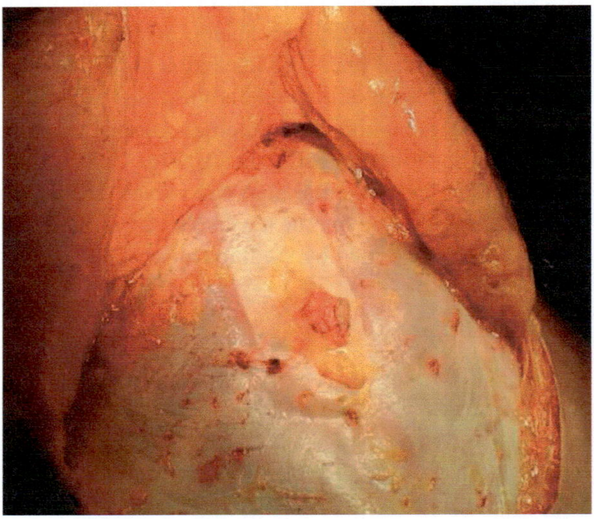

Fig. 1.7 The dehiscence of the linea alba

are, however, more concentrated in the anterior lamina, followed by the posterior lamina, while the middle lamina contains the least [8]. Higher concentrations of elastic fibres in the caudal, anterior, and lateral parts of the linea alba may be an adaptation to more forces in these areas as a consequence of the erectness of the trunk.

Below the umbilicus, the linea alba is weaker due to the absence of the third layers coming from the rectus muscles. During post-pregnancy the upper part is the most affected [8]. With age the linea alba dehisces, reaching 10 mm at 45 years of age and 15 mm after 45 years [7] (Figs. 1.7 and 1.8).

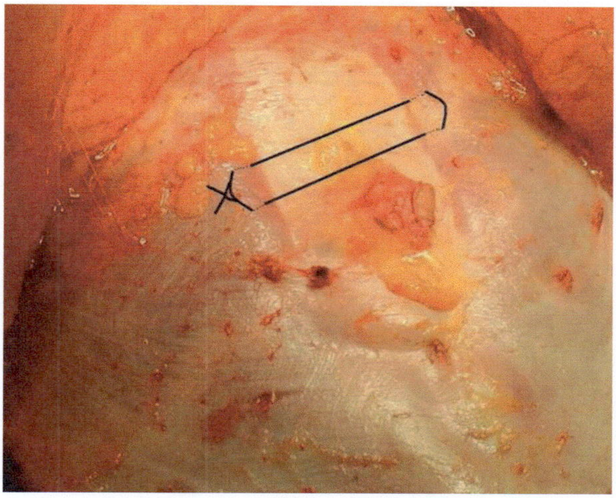

Fig. 1.8 Any suture on the abdominal muscle fascia must be placed perpendicular to the linea alba for a better hold

1.5.2 Rectus Muscle

The rectus is a long, strap-like vertical muscle lying on either side of the midline. The upper part is attached to the external part of the costal cartilages and the xiphoid process, and it ends in the lower abdomen, with insertions into the pubis and symphysis. Superiorly, the rectus is wide at 15 cm, broad, and thin, gradually becoming narrow (7 cm) and thick inferiorly. Segmentation of each rectus muscle occurs through tendinous intersections that attach the rectus muscle with the anterior layer of the rectus sheath. In 80 % of people, there is a small triangular muscle, called the pyramidalis, located anterior to the inferior part of the rectus. This muscle assists in tensing the linea alba.

It is interesting to note that the number of intersections of this muscle appears to have decreased through evolutional history: 12 in horses, 6 in gorillas, and 4 in men [7]. This shows the decreased need of the reinforcement in erected position. The rectus sheath has contributions from all three abdominal muscles' aponeuroses inferior to the umbilicus. The anterior sheath superior to the umbilicus is composed only of aponeuroses from the external and internal abdominal muscles. The transversalis aponeurosis does not assist with the formation of the anterior sheath at this level (Fig. 1.9).

In effect, the internal oblique aponeurosis splits, allowing one layer to pass anteriorly and another one posteriorly to the rectus muscle. The anterior layer will then join with the external oblique aponeurosis to form the anterior wall of the rectus sheath. The anterior sheath can be considered a composite of all three aponeurotic layers at a variable level below the umbilicus. The posterior sheath can be similarly described in relation to the umbilicus. Superior to the umbilicus, the posterior sheath consists of contributions from both the aponeuroses of the internal oblique and the transversus abdominis. Inferior to the umbilicus, the external

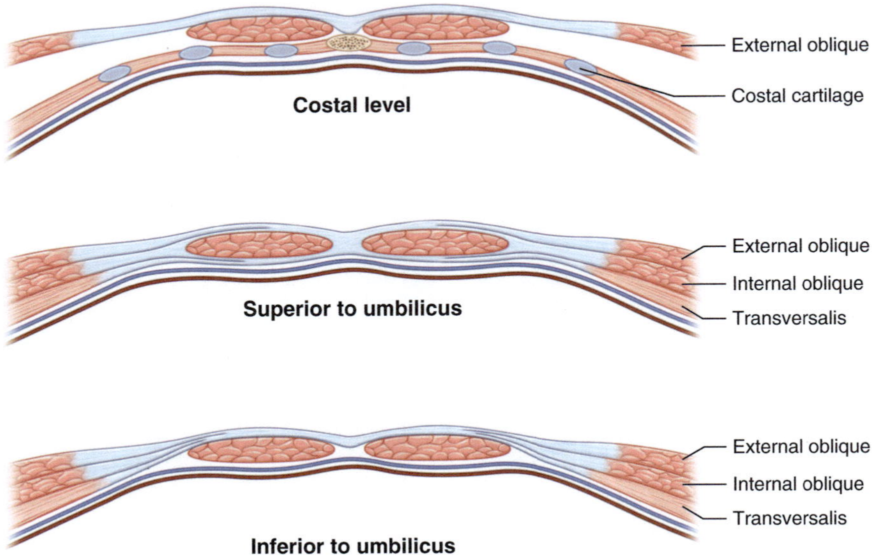

Fig. 1.9 The axial anatomy of linea alba and fascial system at different levels

abdominal aponeurosis does not contribute to the formation of the posterior rectus sheath.

The arcuate line is defined by the most inferior extension of the posterior sheath forming a crescent-shaped border. In the midline, fibres of the anterior and posterior sheaths interlace forming the linea alba. It is now understood that mechanical forces acting here contribute to the formation of epigastric hernias [9].

The ratio of collagen types I and III in the composition of the aponeurosis is a genetic condition, and there is also a change in this in relation to age. With age, the ratio of type I to type III changes in favour of type III which is less elastic and has less capacity to absorb water. Thus, it could be claimed that the aponeurosis becomes weaker and vulnerable with age.

Another factor that may play a role in the correction of the musculoaponeurotic layer is the level of collagen deposits in muscles. Deposits of collagen within the muscles (types I, III, IV, and V) are located in the epimysium, perimysium, and endomysium [10].

With age, there is also an increase in the total number of fibres, which causes the muscles to become less flexible and pliable. This may increase resistance to mobilization of the muscles during the correction of abdominal deformities. Furthermore, it is important to stress that there is a relationship between the size of the musculoaponeurotic deformity and skin excess on the abdomen [4, 10].

Collagen fibres of the rectus fascia after leaving the line alba to medial go with an angle which varies and tends, with age, to end in a horizontal line.

1.5.3 Pyramidalis Muscle

The pyramidalis is a small triangular muscle located anterior to the inferior aspect of rectus abdominis that is absent in about 20 % of the population. The pyramidalis originates from the pubis inferior to the insertion of the rectus abdominis and inserts into the linea alba inferior to the umbilicus to assist in stabilization of the abdominal wall [2].

1.5.4 External Oblique Muscle

This is the most superficial lateral muscle and the largest and thickest of the three flat muscles of the abdomen. The muscle arises from the lowermost eight ribs posteriorly to interdigitate with both the serratus anterior and latissimus dorsi muscles and courses inferior-medially, attaching by means of its aponeurosis centrally at the linea alba. Inferiorly, the external oblique aponeurosis folds back upon itself and forms the inguinal ligament between the anterior superior iliac spine and the pubic tubercle [11].

1.5.5 Internal Oblique Muscle

The internal oblique muscle originates from the anterior portion of iliac crest, lateral half to two-thirds of inguinal ligament, and posterior aponeurosis of the transversus abdominis muscle. The fibres run superiorly–anteriorly at right angles to the external oblique and insert on the cartilages of the lower four ribs [11].

These muscle fibres are differently oriented in the upper and lower parts. The Spiegel line is at the transition of the muscular and aponeurotic parts of the muscle. This weak line can cause lateral hernias [7]. If required, lateral tightening must be done at this line and at the internal oblique level. The aponeurotic part fuses with the opposed muscle aponeurosis in the middle to form the linea alba. This fusion is absent in the lower quarter of the linea alba.

1.5.6 Transversalis Muscle (Transversus Abdominis)

The muscle transversalis is the deepest muscle with horizontally oriented fibres and has a very important role to play in expiration. These muscles arise from the inner surface of the 7th–12th costal cartilages, the iliac crest, and the lateral third of the inguinal ligament. These fibres course medially to the lateral border of the rectus muscle. The end of the muscle fibres and the beginning of aponeurosis is called the linea semilunaris. The aponeurosis fuses to the posterior rectus fascia [4] (Fig. 1.10).

Things to Remember

- Linea alba strongly attaches to the sternum to prevent any hyperextension of the vertebral structures.
- With age the linea alba dehisces, reaching 10 mm at 45 years of age and 15 mm after 45 years.
- With age, the ratio of type I to type III changes in favour of type III which is less elastic and has less capacity to absorb water. Thus, it could be claimed that the aponeurosis becomes weaker and vulnerable with age.
- With age, there is also an increase in the total number of fibres, which causes the muscles to become less flexible and pliable. This may increase resistance to mobilization of the muscles during the correction of abdominal deformities.
- The Spiegel line is at the transition of the muscular and aponeurotic parts of the muscle. This weak line can cause lateral hernias.

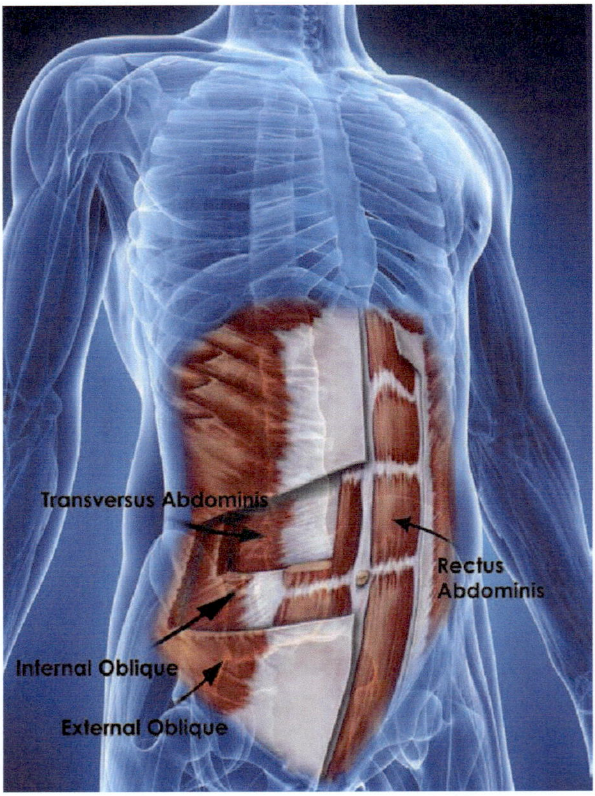

Fig. 1.10 Anterior and lateral abdominal muscles (Pulikkottil et al. [20])

1.6 Abdominal Blood Supply

Three major arterial branches supply blood to either side of the anterior abdominal wall which includes two branches of the external iliac artery and a branch of the internal thoracic artery. The inferior epigastric artery which is a branch of the external iliac artery travels within the transversalis fascia until it reaches the arcuate line where it pierces the rectus sheath. The second branch of the external iliac artery, the deep circumflex iliac artery, runs parallel to the inguinal ligament between the transversus abdominis and internal oblique muscles. The superior epigastric artery, the terminal branch of the internal thoracic artery, enters the rectus sheath superiorly [9] (Fig. 1.11).

The posterior intercostal arteries (which accompany the intercostal nerves) supply the three-ply muscles in the lateral part of the anterior abdominal wall and in this function are reinforced by the lumbar arteries, which are branches of the abdominal aorta [1].

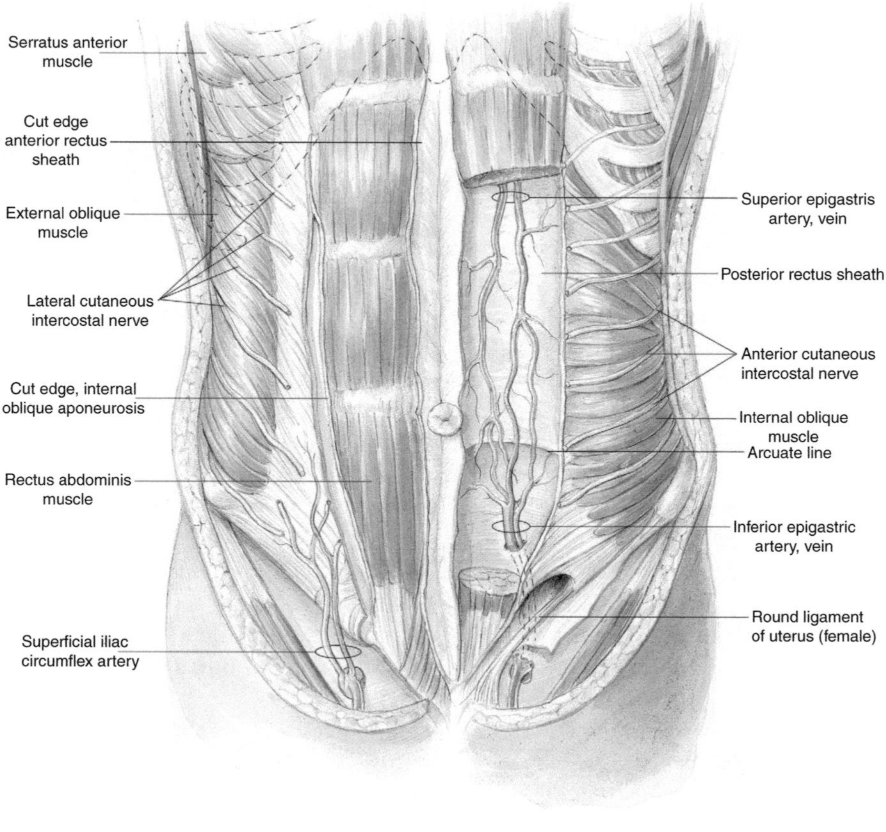

Fig. 1.11 Blood supply – anterior abdominal wall (Ahluwalia et al. [9])

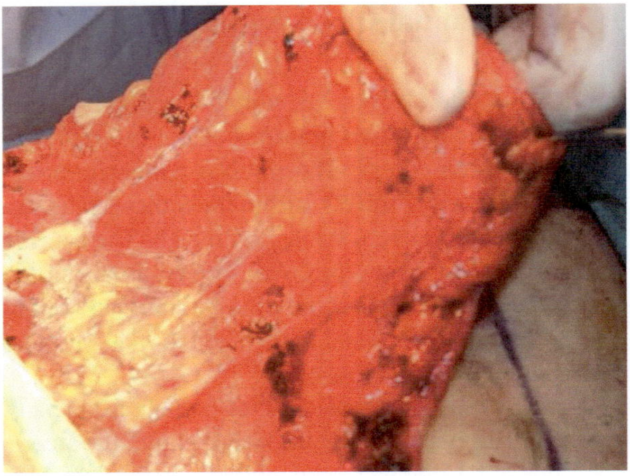

Fig. 1.12 Perforator arteries from rectus muscle (sub-umbilical level)

The rectus abdominis has a dual blood supply. The upper half of the muscle is supplied by the superior epigastric artery (a branch of the internal thoracic artery). The artery enters the rectus abdominis alongside the xiphisternal junction with its companion veins. The lower half of the rectus abdominis is supplied by the deep inferior epigastric artery, a branch of the external iliac artery. Myocutaneous rotation flaps may be fashioned using either the upper or lower halves of the rectus abdominis muscle [1].

The abdominal wall receives its blood supply from direct cutaneous vessels and musculocutaneous perforating vessels [12]. The wall of the arteries perforating the rectus muscle contains more elastic fibres than average. This allows these vessels to keep their perfusion capacity between two gliding tissues: the rectus sheath and deep adipose tissue (Fig. 1.12).

If torn by blunt dissection, these arteries can escape into the rectus fascia and cause intramuscular bleeding, which can lead to long-term pain after abdominoplasty. In obese patients the distribution of these arteries is severely altered.

The deep perforator arteries supply the deep adipose tissues. Superficial adipose tissue is supplied by the arteries from the superficial arterial system. Late lipolyses occurring after abdominoplasty can be explained by the total undermining of the flap from the deep muscular perforated arteries and partial necrosis in the deep fatty tissues [7].

The umbilicus receives blood flow from the surrounding subdermal plexus. In addition, there are three distinct additional sources: the right and left deep inferior epigastric arteries, the ligamentum teres, and the median umbilical ligament. The deep inferior epigastric artery is the dominant blood supplier to the umbilicus.

The umbilicus is more at risk during abdominoplasty performed on a morbidly obese individual because it is elongated and the vascular anatomy is potentially distorted. Shortening the umbilicus by resecting the distal portion may be advantageous in preserving the viability of the umbilicus in these situations [13].

1.7 Lymphatic System of the Abdomen

The lymphatic channels reside within the sub-scarpal fat layer superficial to the anterior rectus sheath. Soft tissue lymphatics above the umbilicus drain to axillary lymph nodes, while those below the umbilicus drain to the superficial inguinal lymph nodes. It has been reported that preservation of the subfascial lymphatic system diminishes the accumulation of serious post-abdominoplasty fluid and the need for drains. There are many publications discussing the advantages of this technique [6–8, 10, 14–17].

1.8 Abdominal Nerves

Cutaneous innervation of the abdominal wall is consistent with the segmental dermatomal pattern. The anterior and lateral cutaneous branches of the ventral rami of the 7th–12th intercostal nerves and the ventral rami of the first and second lumbar nerves have important sensory and motor functions [9] (Fig. 1.13).

1.8.1 Thoracoabdominal Nerves

The lateral cutaneous branches of intercostal and subcostal nerves supply sensation to the lateral portion of the abdomen. The anterior branches of the intercostal and subcostal nerves supply sensation to the midline abdomen.

These nerves are deep structures. Taking small amounts of fat from a periumbilical area is permitted by superficial local anaesthetics, but in the long-term, patients complain about pain in this area. It is advised to deeply inject the anaesthetics into the fascia to obtain long-term comfort. This is because terminal nerves from the iliohypogastric and ilioinguinal nerves are also supplying the periumbilical area.

1.8.2 Iliohypogastric Nerve (T12, L1)

Iliohypogastric nerve innervates the skin and soft tissue over the iliac crest and lateral thigh. Nerve entrapment during the rectus anterior sheath plication has been reported. Persistent lower abdominal wall pain occurring postoperatively, despite negative gastrointestinal and/or gynecologic pathology, should alert the surgeon to the possibility of iliohypogastric or ilioinguinal nerve entrapment. Diagnosis can be made if there is subsequent relief after nerve block and treatment consists of

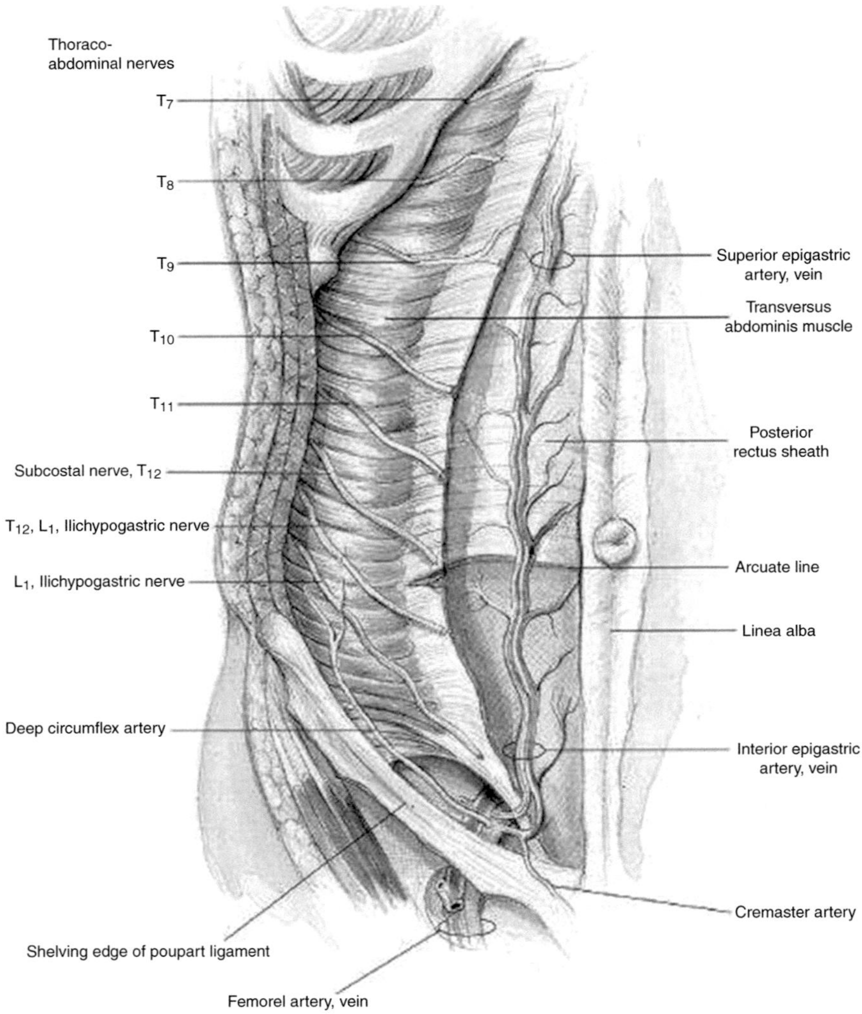

Fig. 1.13 Nerve supply of the anterior abdominal wall (Ahluwalia et al. [9])

performing a neurectomy at the level of the retroperitoneum to avoid recurrent painful neuromas [18].

1.8.3 Ilioinguinal Nerve (L1)

The ilioinguinal nerve innervates lower abdominal skin. Coursing from the mons superiorly, these nerves are often divided bilaterally during caesarean sections, and many post-caesarean section patients have numbness of the lower abdominal skin. This may be an advantage for post-operative comfort.

1.8.4 Genitofemoral Nerve

This nerve exits the muscular fascia at the level of the inguinal ligament in the middle of its length. The surgeon shall preserve the lateral femoral cutaneous branch, which innervates the anterior thigh. The damage to this branch results in chronic numbness of the anterior thigh, which can be very annoying because of the difference between the sensitivity perception on the left and right sides [6].

Things to Remember

- Shortening the umbilicus by resecting the distal portion may be advantageous in preserving the viability of the umbilicus in these situations.
- Persistent lower abdominal wall pain occurring postoperatively, despite negative gastrointestinal and/or gynecologic pathology, should alert the surgeon to the possibility of iliohypogastric or ilioinguinal nerve entrapment.
- The surgeon shall preserve the lateral femoral cutaneous branch, which innervates the anterior thigh.

References

1. Mahadevan V. Anatomy of the anterior abdominal wall and groin. Surgery (Oxford). 2003;21(2):25–7.
2. Grevious MA, Cohen M, Shah SR, Rodriguez P. Structural and functional anatomy of the abdominal wall. Clin Plast Surg. 2006;33(2):169–79, v.
3. Cunningham SC, Rosson GD, Lee RH, et al. Localization of the arcuate line from surface anatomic landmarks: a cadaveric study. Ann Plast Surg. 2004;53(2):129–31.
4. Lancerotto L, Stecco C, Macchi V, et al. Layers of the abdominal wall: anatomical investigation of subcutaneous tissue and superficial fascia. Surg Radiol Anat. 2011;33(10):835–42.
5. Lockwood TE. Superficial fascial system (SFS) of the trunk and extremities: a new concept. Plast Reconstr Surg. 1991;87:1009–18.

6. Costa-Ferreira A, Rodrigues-Pereira P, Rebelo M, Vásconez LO, Amarante J. Morphometric study (macroscopic and microscopic) of the lower abdominal wall. Plast Reconstr Surg. 2014;134(6):1313–22.
7. Caix P. Anatomie de la paroi abdominal. Ann Chir Plast Esthet. 1999;44(4):289–311.
8. Rath AM, Attali P, Dumas JL, Goldlust D, Zhang J, Chevrel JP. The abdominal linea alba: an anatomic-radiologic and biomechanical study. Surg Radiol Anat. 1996;18:281.
9. Ahluwalia HS, Burger JP, Quinn TH. Anatomy of anterior abdominal wall. Operatives Tech In Plast Surg. 2004;6(3):147–55.
10. Monkhouse WS, Khalique A. Variations in the composition of the human rectus sheath: a study of the anterior abdominal wall. J Anat. 1986;145:61–6.
11. Moore KL, Dalley AF. Clinically oriented anatomy. 4th ed. Philadelphia: Lippincott Williams & Wilkins; 1999.
12. Nahai F, Brown RG, Vasconez LO. Blood supply to the abdominal wall as related to planning abdominal incisions. Am Surg. 1976;42(9):691–5.
13. Nahai F. Anatomical considerations in abdominoplasty. Clin Plast Surg. 2010;37(3):407–14.
14. Le Louarn C. Partial subfascial abdominoplasty. Aesthetic Plast Surg. 1996;20:123–7.
15. Costa-Ferreira A, Rebelo M, Va'sconez LO, Amarante J. Scarpa fascia preservation during abdominoplasty: a prospective study. Plast Reconstr Surg. 2010;125:1232–9.
16. Fang RC, Lin SJ, Mustoe TA. Abdominoplasty flap elevation in a more superficial plane: decreasing the need for drains. Plast Reconstr Surg. 2010;125:677–82.
17. Richter D. The scarpa lift, Paper presented at: 39th annual meeting of the German Society of plastic, reconstructive and aesthetic surgeons; Oct 2008; Germany.
18. Liszka TG, Dellon AL, Manson PN. Iliohypogastric nerve entrapment following abdominoplasty. Plast Reconstr Surg. 1994;93:181–4.
19. Moore KL. Clinically oriented anatomy. Baltimore: Williams & Wilkins; 1992.
20. Pulikkottil BJ, Pezeshk RA, Daniali LN, Bailey SH, Mapula S, Hoxworth RE. Lateral Abdominal Wall Defects: The Importance of Anatomy and Technique for a Successful Repair. Plast Reconstr Surg Glob Open. 2015;3:e481. doi:10.1097/GOX.0000000000000439.

Chapter 2
Anesthesia and Algology in Abdominal Surgery

Ibrahim Ozdilmac

2.1 Introduction

Whether minor or major, completing any surgical intervention with minimum or no complication is the most important desire of the surgeon and the patient. Sometimes, the realization of this desire may not be enough on its own. Patients' contentment and acceptance of the procedure performed may be more important than even minor complications.

In this respect, one of the factors that may affect the perception of a successful surgery is to provide a satisfactory anesthesia and analgesia. This is important for the satisfaction of the patient as well as the surgeon. This can be achieved to a great extent with careful analgesic assessment beginning from the preoperative evaluation to the postoperative analgesia process and with the application of personally adapted anesthesia methods.

Anesthesia applications pertaining to abdominal wall surgery are diversified, and the appropriate method is selected in accordance with the medical condition of the patient. Indications of these operations include cosmetics, conditions after abdominal trauma, excessive weight loss after bariatric surgery, ventral hernia, postinfectious cases, and abdominal wall disorders [1]. Although the number of patients in each of these categories is not known exactly, around 164,000 abdominoplasty operations were performed in 2014, and it ranks fourth in terms of frequency among all cosmetic procedures according to the national cosmetic surgery data of American Aesthetic Plastic Surgery Association [2].

Since the 1970s the number of surgical interventions in outpatient centers out of hospitals has gradually increased, leading to approximately 70 % of elective surgeries being performed in outpatient centers [3]. In parallel, more than 50 % of esthetic

I. Ozdilmac
Anaesthetist, Florence Nightingale Hospital Istanbul, Cemil Aslan Güder Sok. No: 8
Gayrettepe, Istanbul, Turkey
e-mail: iozdilmac@yahoo.com

K.T. Tiryaki (ed.), *Inverse Abdominoplasty*, DOI 10.1007/978-3-319-39310-0_2

plastic surgeons prefer performing interventions in appropriate office conditions [4]. Although many factors contribute to a preference to ambulatory surgery, the main factor is an economic advantage [5]. To reduce perioperative morbidity and mortality, it is safe to have advanced monitoring capability and to adopt the monitoring standards of the American Society of Anesthesiologists (ASA) [6]. Developments in pharmacology have helped to reduce morbidity through the use of anesthetic agents with short-term and rapid effects [7]. Ambulatory anesthesia became an official subbranch of anesthesia upon the foundation of the Society of Ambulatory Anesthesia (SAMBA) in 1984. After the evaluation of 1.1 million outpatients, the mortality rate after ambulatory anesthesia was demonstrated to be 1.5/100,000 [8]. No mortality occurred in the 319,000 patients monitored in accordance with ASA standards [9].

In most of the surgeries out of hospitals, the surgeon has an important role in medical decisions on procedures pertaining to anesthesia. In general, the surgeon makes the final decision on procurement of personnel, postoperative pain treatment, and adopted discharge criteria as well as the location of the surgery, degree of preoperative assessment, type of anesthesia, and care and monitorization of the patient. If the surgeon prefers to undertake the anesthesia, he/she has to know the latest standards in anesthesia practice and has to abide by the same standards applied by the anesthetist. One should not feel comfortable considering the decrease in mortality and morbidity in anesthesia and should pay attention to accreditation in centers out of hospitals [10].

Things to Remember: Box 2.1

- An anesthesia method appropriate for a person together with a careful and cautious anamnesis increases success and satisfaction.
- ASA criteria must be applied for a safe procedure.

2.2 Centers Where Surgeries Take Place

The surgeon decides on and is responsible for determination of the center where the procedure will be applied in accordance with the operation. These centers can be reviewed under three main categories:

2.2.1 Under Hospital Conditions

Things to Remember: Box 2.2

- Ambulatory surgery decreases surgical costs.
- However, a suitable monitorization is sine qua non.

(a) Inpatient
(b) Outpatient

2.2.2 In Independent Surgical Centers

Things to Remember: Box 2.3

- Accreditation is essential in outpatient centers.
- The main purpose of final decision on procedures is to ensure patient safety.

(a) Requiring short-term follow-up
(b) Not requiring short-term follow-up

2.2.3 Under Office Conditions

2.2.3.1 Prepared Operational Rooms

Each of these preferences has different advantages and disadvantages. Surgical procedures performed under accredited office conditions are economic and useful as well as proving to be safer when compared to surgical procedures performed in other centers [11]. Regardless of the type of anesthesia or selected center, the operational room must be fully equipped and meet the monitoring criteria adopted by the ASA, such as having appropriate resuscitation equipment and drugs. The surgical center must have personnel who are educated in patient care and can assist the surgeon when necessary. Emergency protocols must be determined, and there must be a contracted hospital and laboratory available when necessary [12]. As a result, the main purpose in decision taking pertaining to the procedures to be performed is to ensure patient safety.

One of the most important factors for successful surgical results is the personnel assisting the surgeon. The person responsible for the selection of personnel to work in operating rooms under office conditions is the surgeon.

In small-area liposuctions applied with tumescent technique, the surgeon may prefer to perform using only local anesthesia without parenteral sedation [13]. However, many surgeons demand parenteral sedation and analgesia in addition to local anesthesia. Providing both patient and surgeon satisfaction as mentioned in the beginning finds its place exactly at this point. If parenteral sedation is preferred, licensed and experienced staff should monitor the patient during the operation. There has to be a personnel with "Advanced Cardiac Life Support" certificate in the center where the surgery takes place, and the other healthcare personnel working in the operational room have to be educated in "Basic Life Support" [14].

Things to Remember: Box 2.4

- Responsibility pertaining to the procedure to be performed and selection of the personnel belongs to the surgeon.
- An experienced and certified personnel will facilitate the work of the surgeon.

Table 2.1 Guidelines for preoperative testing in healthy patients (ASA I–II)

Age	Test
12–40[a]	CBC (complete blood count)
40–60	CBC, EKG
60↑	CBC, EKG, BUN, CXR, glucose

Adapted from Shiffmann [16]

[a]A pregnancy test is suggested for potentially childbearing females

2.3 Preoperative Assessment

As stated in the introduction part, the determination of the appropriate anesthesia method for each patient is essential for satisfactory results for both the patient and the surgeon. This can be achieved with a careful preoperative assessment and preparation phase.

Accurate preoperative assessment and preparation increases the patient's confidence in the surgeon as well as minimizing the perioperative risks for the patient by reducing unnecessary time losses and thus costs. The medical conditions of about 90 % of patients can be assessed simply with the information obtained in anamnesis. An information form to be prepared for checking the information obtained and facilitating to contact the patient is highly effective. Thanks to the questions in this form, it is possible to obtain satisfactory information on the medical history of the patient, surgical procedures undergone and applied anesthesia types, adverse effects arising in the former anesthesia or with the drugs used, diet applied due to obesity and agents used for this purpose, eating habits, and allergic conditions [15].

Tests that must be applied preoperatively may vary depending on the patient's age and information obtained from the patient. Table 2.1 demonstrates a general approach for healthy patients who do not use any drugs [16]. Additional tests may also be required depending on the risk factors and medical conditions of the patient. For a patient defining chest pain and shortness of breath despite a young age, an EKG and chest x-ray will be appropriate. Similarly, appropriate tests must be applied in cases of urine findings, hepatitis history, diabetes, or thyroid disease.

Certain risk factors such as undiagnosed hypertension, cardiac arrhythmia, or bronchial asthma can be detected with preoperative physical examination. Risk assessment in terms of intubation by considering the head and neck structure of the patient is essential. Preoperative assessment of the patient by an anesthetist is an appropriate and necessary approach for both planning the anesthesia to be applied to the patient and minimizing the perioperative risks.

Many authors agree on common points in morbidity and mortality: performing more than one procedure at a time, prolonged surgeries, significant blood loss, and wide invasive surgeries have increased perioperative complication risks. In order to minimize the risk of cardiopulmonary complications and optimize tissue perfusion in liposuctions, the aspired amount must be less than 5 % of the body weight and 30 % of the body surface, as a rule [17].

Table 2.2 Current definitions (no change) and examples (new) [18][a]

ASA PS classification	Definition	Examples include but not limited to
ASA I	A normal healthy patient	Healthy, non-smoking, no or minimal alcohol use
ASA II	A patient with mild systemic disease	Mild diseases only without substantive functional limitations. Examples include (but not limited to) current smoker, social alcohol drinker, pregnancy, obesity (30< BMI <40), well-controlled DM/HTN, mild lung disease
ASA III	A patient with severe systemic disease	Substantive functional limitations; one or more moderate to severe diseases. Examples include (but not limited to) poorly controlled DM or HTN, COPD, morbid obesity (BMI ≥40), active hepatitis, alcohol dependence or abuse, implanted pacemaker, moderate reduction of ejection fraction, ESRD undergoing regularly scheduled dialysis, premature infant PCA <60 weeks, history (>3 months) of MI, TIA, or CAD/stents
ASA IV	A patient with severe systemic disease that is a constant threat to life	Examples include (but not limited to) recent (<3 months) MI, CVA, TIA, or CAD/stents; ongoing cardiac ischemia or severe valve dysfunction; severe reduction of ejection fraction; sepsis; DIC; ARD; or ESRD not undergoing regularly scheduled dialysis
ASA V	A moribund patient who is not expected to survive without the operation	Examples include (but not limited to) ruptured abdominal/thoracic aneurysm, massive trauma, intracranial bleed with mass effect, ischemic bowel in the face of significant cardiac pathology, or multiple organ/system dysfunction
ASA VI	A declared brain-dead patient whose organs are being removed for donor purposes	

[a]The addition of "E" denotes emergency surgery: (An emergency is defined as existing when a delay in treatment of the patient would lead to a significant increase in the threat to life or body part.)

The most common method in preoperative risk evaluation is the ASA (American Society of Anesthesiologists) classification. Table 2.2 demonstrates the ASA classification which was extended and accepted in 2014 [18].

Things to Remember: Box 2.5

Risk Factors

- Undiagnosed hypertension
- Cardiac arrhythmia
- Bronchial asthma
- More than one procedure at a time
- Prolonged surgeries
- Significant blood loss
- Wide surface-invasive surgeries

Things to Remember: Box 2.6
- Preoperative evaluation forms provide very essential information.
- ASA classification must be performed.

Things to Remember: Box 2.7
- The amount aspired in liposuctions which is less than 5 % of body weight and less than 30 % of body surface as a rule reduces complications.

Cardiac diseases are associated with serious complications leading to perioperative mortality. One should be particularly careful in assessment of asymptomatic patients with risk factors such as obesity, diabetes, hypertension, hyperlipidemia, cigarette use, or serious cardiac diseases in the family. While planning anesthesia for patients with significant cardiac diseases, it is preferable to perform the surgical procedure under hospital conditions rather than office conditions. For any effective surgery to be performed after a myocardial infarction (MI), the surgery must be planned for at least 6 months later [19]. Hemodynamic stability must be ensured in order to prevent perioperative ischemic attacks.

Obesity is associated with risk factors such as hypertension, coronary arterial disease, hyperlipidemia, diabetes, obstructive sleep apnea (OSA), and degenerative disc disease. Perioperative pulmonary emboli risk is considerably high in morbid obesity. Obesity attended by any one of these risk factors increases the complication risk in anesthesia [20]. In the obesity assessment of the patient, body mass index (BMI kg/m^2) and waist-hip ratio are used. If the waist circumference is longer than 102 cm for male patients and longer than 89 cm for female patients, they are accepted as high risk in terms of obesity-related diseases. Patients with BMI values over 30 are evaluated as obese, and patients with BMI values over 35 are evaluated as morbidly obese [21]. Hypertension is very common in these patients and must be under control during operation. If there are symptoms or findings pertaining to heart failure or coronary artery disease in morbidly obese patients, it is appropriate to apply advanced tests (such as echocardiography, dobutamine stress test, etc.) to evaluate myocardial damage. In patients having undergone bariatric surgery before abdominoplasty, an additional careful assessment must be performed in terms of nutrition and vitamin deficiencies [1].

Things to Remember: Box 2.8
- BMI >30→obese
- BMI >35→morbid obese
- Attention for additional diseases

Things to Remember: Box 2.9

For male patients

- If WC (waist circumference) >102 cm

For female patients

- If WC >89 cm, then they are in high-risk category which means they might have an obesity-related disease.

Hypertension is accepted by many authors as a disease that must be stabilized before an operation. Perioperative cardiovascular complications such as ischemia can be addressed, and thus morbidity and mortality can be reduced [22]. In patients undergoing hypertension treatment, drugs must be used until the morning of the operation day due to rebound hypertension risk. An exception to this case is angiotensin-converting enzyme (ACE) inhibitors. Since this group of drugs may lead to hypotension during anesthesia induction, they must be ceased before operation [23].

Diabetes Mellitus is a case increasing surgical mortality particularly when it is not regulated. It can increase the tendency toward many end-organ diseases such as cardiovascular, renal, or different wound healing [24]. Keeping in mind that silent myocardial ischemia incidence is high in diabetic patients, necessary care must be provided in preoperative assessment [25]. In type 1 or type 2 diabetic patients, the purpose is firstly to prevent hypoglycemia in perioperative treatment. For this purpose, blood sugar follow-ups must be performed carefully beginning from the morning of the operation day until the patient is discharged, and interventions must be performed with appropriate procedures when necessary.

Pulmonary diseases cover conditions that can affect pulmonary functions during operation and are widely encountered. The most frequent conditions include upper respiratory tract infections, chronic bronchitis, chronic obstructive pulmonary disease, bronchial asthma, and a cigarette habit. In cases of upper respiratory tract diseases, operations must be postponed until symptoms such as coughing, fever, expectorating, and shaking fully dissipate, particularly in patients for whom general anesthesia is considered. In a prospective study, it was demonstrated that postoperative pulmonary complication risk increases by approximately sixfold in smoking patients. It was detected that reducing smoking within 1 month before the surgery is not associated with any decrease in postoperative pulmonary complication risk [26]. Management of asthma patients with success can be achieved by determining whether they are in attack or not via a careful anamnesis and physical examination and by an appropriate intervention. If the asthma is under control, it does not constitute any additional risk in terms of perioperative complications. In contrast, in cases of inadequately controlled asthma, perioperative complication risk is almost always present [27]. Therefore, treatment of asthma patients must be continued until the surgery, and patients must be educated regarding postoperative airway exercises.

Things to Remember: Box 2.10

- If a patient had a myocardial infarction, any elective surgery must be planned for at least 6 months after that.

Things to Remember: Box 2.11

- Hypertension, diabetes, and asthma must be regulated preoperatively.
- Treatments must be continued until surgical day (except for ACE inhibitors).

Obstructive Sleep Apnea (OSA) can be defined as a sleep disorder where respiration stops for five times or more within an hour of sleep, during more than 10 s despite respiratory efforts, and characterized by 4 % or more decrease in arterial saturation [28]. Many drugs from sedative, hypnotic, or narcotic-analgesic group which are used during anesthesia increase airway obstruction risk and lead to respiratory depression particularly in patients with OSA. In patients with severe OSA whose apnea-hypopnea index is higher than 30 in an hour, the desaturation possibility of the patient during anesthesia induction is evaluated as very high [29]. Patients with OSA generally use home-type CPAP (continuous positive airway pressure) masks to reduce symptoms. If the CPAP required for the patient is more than 10 cm H2O, ventilation with mask can much possibly be difficult [30].

2.4 Anesthesia Methods in Abdominoplasty

Anesthetic approaches can be reviewed under two categories as general anesthesia and regional anesthesia. Apart from these, sedative and nonsedative local anesthesia can also be applied in minor invasive surgeries over small areas.

2.4.1 General Anesthesia

General anesthesia is a particularly appropriate choice for those patients whose narcotic and sedative drug toleration is high, who suffer from extreme anxiety, and who will undergo major surgeries. The purpose of general anesthesia is to achieve a soft induction, to provide a complete and smooth wake-up, and to minimize side effects such as nausea, vomiting, and throat pain. Isoflurane, sevoflurane, and desflurane are the newest inhalation anesthetic agents. They have rapidly become popular since they are safe, protective, and easy to use.

Since the airway reflexes are blocked in general anesthesia, airway control is the most critical issue to which attention must be paid. The purpose of airway management is to maintain an open airway, to provide adequate ventilation, and to prevent aspiration of the stomach content. In obese patients, total pulmonary capacity, expiratory reserve volume (ERV), and functional residual capacity (FRC) decrease depending on the BMI increase. Thus, tendency toward arterial hypoxemia has increased due to ventilation-perfusion inconsistency and right-left shunt [31]. This is clearer in the supine position, and one must be careful since hypoxemia and desaturation may develop rapidly in anesthesia induction.

Things to Remember: Box 2.12

- Obese patient ventilation is difficult under general anesthesia, and desaturation develops rapidly.
- Attention for aspiration of stomach content.

2.4.2 Regional Anesthesia

Regional anesthesia may be applied in different ways: complete regional anesthesia without any additional anesthesia, regional anesthesia applied together with a mild sedation, and regional interventions applied to achieve postoperative pain control in procedures performed under general anesthesia.

In patients who will undergo abdominal wall surgery, dermatome area from T4 to L1 must be blocked. This region can be anesthetized through epidural or spinal anesthesia. While this method may provide the required anesthesia in the surgical area on its own, it can also be used together with general anesthesia or sedation. Surgical anesthesia is achieved within 5–15 min with spinal anesthesia. Applying the local anesthetic agent directly to cerebrospinal fluid (CSF) ensures rapid start for effect. There is certain recently reported information regarding abdominoplasty surgery performed by using spinal anesthesia under office conditions [32]. Spinal anesthesia can be performed through single-entry technique, or an intrathecal catheter can be placed when the surgery is estimated to last a long time.

In epidural anesthesia, a catheter is placed in the epidural cavity before the dura. The local anesthetic applied from the catheter is diffused from the dura and affects nerve roots. This is an ideal method for both intraoperative anesthesia and continuance of postoperative surgical area analgesia. During the last decade, the use of the combined epidural-spinal technique has been gradually increasing [33]. While surgical anesthesia is rapidly obtained with this method, the availability to intervene to extend the block allows us to adjust the regional block depth. There are certain limitations for patients undergoing spinal, epidural, or combined spinal-epidural anesthesia for abdominoplasty operation. While an effective intraoperative anesthesia is achieved through caudal spreading of local anesthetic, the sensory-motor block formed in lower extremities prevents early mobilization and increases urinary retention. Local anesthetic spreading toward the cranium may lead to paralysis in accessory respiratory muscles including the diaphragm and pressure in respiration. Local anesthetic spreading upward may block spinal cardiac accelerator fibers and thus decrease cardiac output and result in hypotension. Besides, since there is a mobilization restriction in patients undergoing abdominal wall surgery, anticoagulant treatment need must be kept in mind as a protective measure against thromboembolism [1–33]. As a result, regional anesthesia may not be appropriate for every patient undergoing abdominal wall surgery.

2.4.3 Planar Blocks: Transverse Abdominis Plane (TAP) Block

TAP block is a regional anesthesia technique providing analgesia on the frontal abdominal wall up to the parietal peritoneum including the muscles and skin. Compared to modern techniques it is not used much in practice, despite its high-success rate and relatively low-complication risk [34]. Subumbilical anesthesia of the abdominal frontal wall is achieved by applying local anesthetic in a high volume (20 ml) with a special needle together with ultrasound between the internal oblique muscle on lumbar Petit triangle and transverse abdominis muscle. When the oblique subcostal TAP block is added, the whole abdominal frontal wall is anesthetized [1–34].

Postoperative pain treatment is worrisome for both surgeons and patients. In order to achieve a painless postoperative period, many methods such as local anesthetic infiltrations, epidural analgesia, peripheral nerve disorders, and intravenous patient-controlled analgesia (iv-PCA) are used. TAP block takes its place as a safe and effective method that can be applied easily under ultrasound guidance to reduce postoperative pain in lower abdominal region [35]. It is more important for patients with high risks such as obstructive sleep apnea since it reduces the need for postoperative narcotic drugs [35, 36]. In the labeled pictures below, some examples of ultrasound-guided TAP block are shown (Pictures 2.1, 2.2, and 2.3).

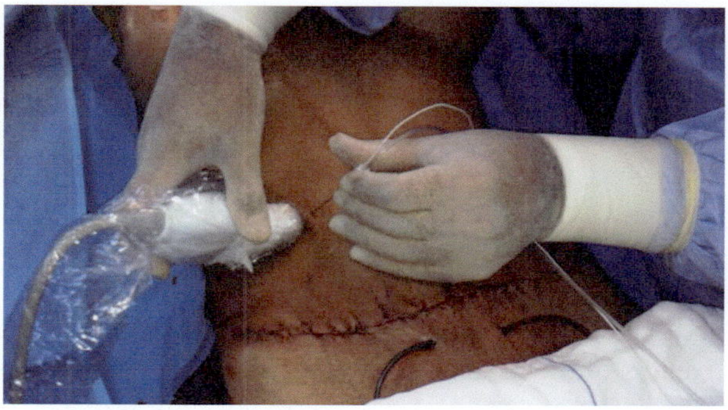

Picture 2.1 Ultrasound-guided TAP block (From the right lumbar Petit triangle)

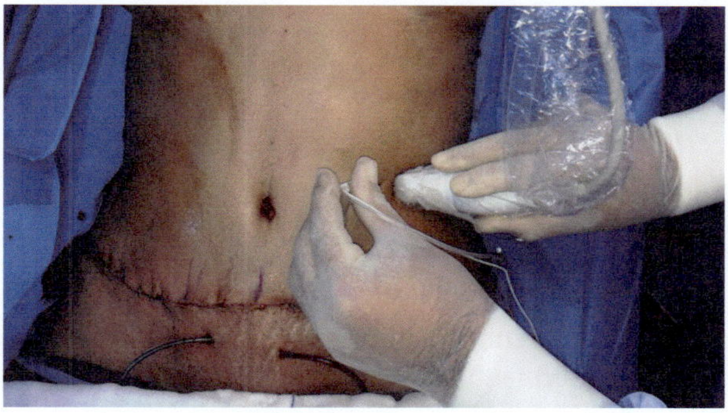

Picture 2.2 Ultrasound-guided TAP block (From the left lumbar Petit triangle)

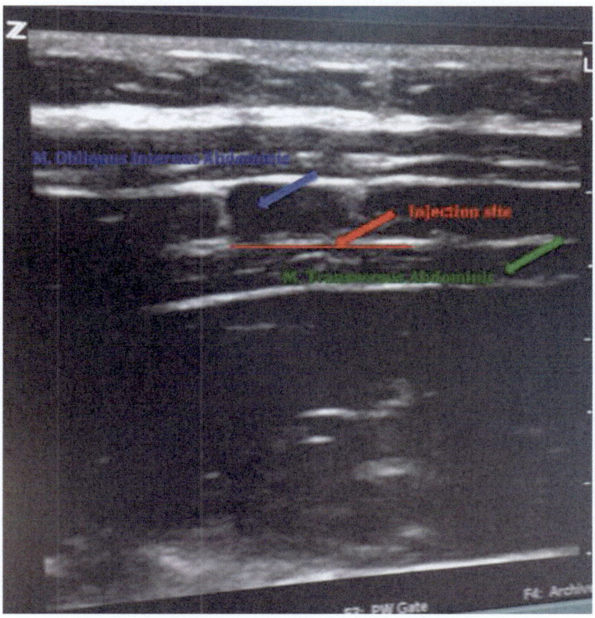

Picture 2.3 Ultrasound vision at TAP block

Things to Remember: Box 2.13

- TAP block is very effective in postoperative analgesia.
- It reduces narcotic needs and provides advantages to OSA patients.

2.4.4 Local Anesthesia

There are many local anesthetics used for infiltrative anesthesia. Safeness and effectiveness of the local anesthetic is the most important point for cosmetic plastic surgeons. The use of local anesthetic not only provides adequate anesthesia after an operation and during procedures applied but also minimizes blood loss and supports postoperative analgesia [37].

The basic pharmacologic effects of all local anesthetics are realized over sodium channels. Sodium entrance into neuron is blocked, and thus axon depolarization is ceased, and the local anesthetic effect begins. In addition to local anesthetic effect, it restricts inflammatory response by reducing the release of inflammatory cytokines from neutrophils, neutrophil adhesion to endothelium, free oxygen radical formation, and edema [38].

Local anesthetics are divided into the two main groups of ester and amid depending on their chemical structures and their characteristics that are demonstrated in Fig. 2.1. Information on the effective time and dose range of the amide group local anesthetics, used widely in infiltration anesthesia, is summarized in Table 2.3.

Undesired conditions such as nerve damage, ecchymosis, hematoma, infection, or pain may occur during local anesthetic injection. The use of small needles, slow injection, and handling tissues kindly may minimize these complications. Any pain arising from pH of the solution can be reduced by adding 1 ml sodium bicarbonate for each 10 ml anesthetic (8.4 %) [39].

Systemic complications can be observed as an allergic response or toxicity associated with local anesthetic. Allergic reactions including urticaria, angioedema, and anaphylaxis can be treated with conservative methods. Toxicity may occur as a result of direct injection of anesthetic to major vessel, exceeding the maximum dose amount, or by a decrease in the metabolism of a drug. Symptoms and findings that may arise in systemic intoxication of local anesthetics are summarized in Fig. 2.2.

Those in the amide group are metabolized with cytochrome P-450 CYP3A4 enzyme in the liver. Drugs inhibiting this enzyme can increase the concentration of local anesthetic [37]. A list of drugs inhibiting cytochrome P-450 CYP3A4 enzyme is provided in Table 2.4.

All local anesthetics except for ropivacaine and cocaine are vasodilators. While preparing local anesthetic solution, adrenaline is used to benefit from its vasoconstrictor effect. Thus, the aim is to reach the highest possible dose by decreasing the passing of the drug to blood. It can be used in concentrations diluted by more than 1/100,000. Cardiac side effects (tachycardia, hypertension, chest pain, etc.) can be

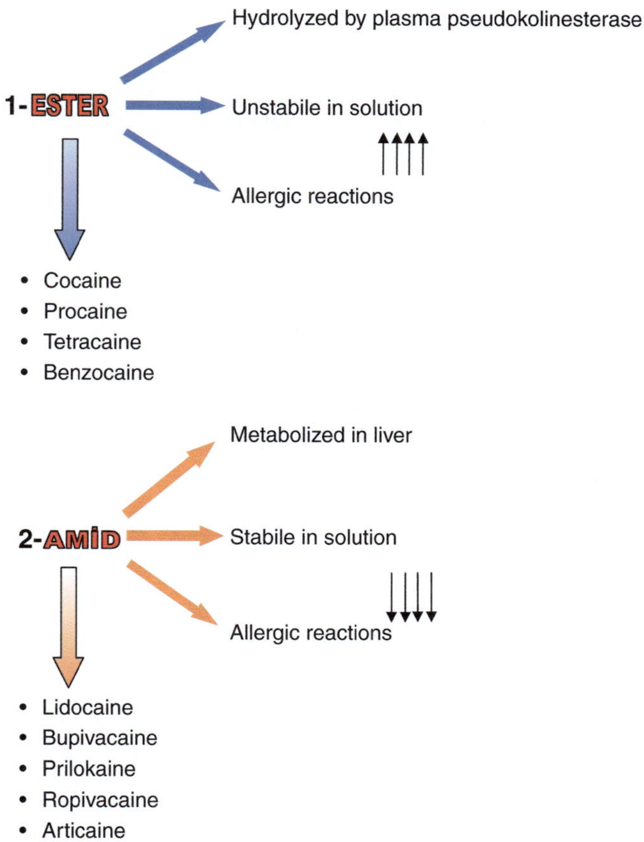

Fig. 2.1 Classification of local anesthetics

treated with vasodilator agents (nitroglycerine, hydralazine, etc.) [37]. It can be kept in mind that the use of adrenaline solution in patients taking monoamine oxidase inhibitor may lead to significant hypertension. Although the maximum dose of adrenaline-lidocaine in routine use is recorded as 7 mg/kg, it can be used in higher doses such as 35–55 mg/kg in tumescent liposuctions [40]. If lidocaine will be used, certain authors suggest not using lidocaine in infiltration solutions of more than 4 L in order to avoid toxicity [41].

High-volume tumescent anesthesia of the abdomen and lower extremities may lead to a decrease in venous flow including deep venous thrombosis and venous stasis. This may increase tissue-clotting factors and increases the pulmonary thromboembolism risk in patients with low mobilization [37]. The use of mechanical compression tools together with a low-molecular-weight heparin is strongly suggested for thrombosis prophylaxis in plastic surgery patients with high risk in terms of venous thromboembolism [42].

Table 2.3 Characteristics of certain local anesthetics used frequently in infiltration anesthesia

Without epinephrine						With epinephrine			
Agent	Concentration (%)	Duration of action (min)	mg/kg total	Total ml	Maximum dose	Duration of action (min)	mg/kg total	Total ml	Maximum dose
Lidocaine	1	30–60	4	300	30	120	7	500	50
Bupivacaine	0.25	120–240	2.5	185	75	180	3	225	90
Ropivacaine	0.2	120–360	2.7	200	8	120–360	2.7	200	80
Etidocaine	0.5	120–180	4.0	300	60	180	5.5	400	80
Mepivacaine	1.0	45–90	4.0	300	30	120	7	500	50

Adapted from Shiffmann [16]

Things to Remember: Box 2.14

- All local anesthetics apart from ropivacaine and cocaine are vasodilators.
- MAO inhibitor + adrenaline solution = hypertension.
- High-volume tumescent anesthesia may lead to a decrease in venous flow and deep venous thrombosis.

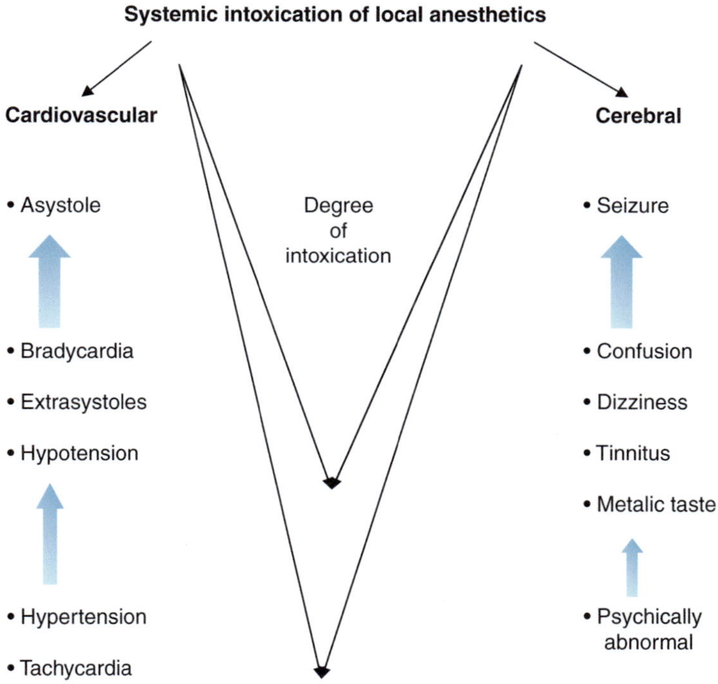

Fig. 2.2 Symptoms and findings that may arise in systemic intoxication of local anesthetics

2.4.5 Sedation-Analgesia

Sedative-analgesic drugs are used in most of abdominoplasties performed under local or regional anesthesia. These drugs aim to reduce anxiety, and state of consciousness and pain sense could prevent the patient from remembering the surgery. Sedation, defined as a decrease in consciousness level as a result of drugs given, can be divided into four main categories. Table 2.5 demonstrates the sedation classification defined by the American Anesthesia Association in October 2014 [43].

Minimal sedation (anxiolytics) is a state where patient can respond to verbal questions normally after the drug is given. Although cognitive functions and physical coordination are reduced, airway reflexes, respiration, and cardiovascular functions are not affected.

Table 2.4 Medications inhibiting cytochrome oxidase P4503A4

Amiodarone	Diltiazem	Isoniazid	Nifedipine	Tetracycline
Atenolol	Erythromycin	Labetalol	Paroxetine	Terfenadine
Carbamazepine	Fluconazole	Ketoconazole	Pentoxifylline	Thyroxine
Cimetidine	Flurazepam	Methylprednisolone	Propofol	Timolol
Clarithromycin	Fluoxetine	Midazolam	Propranolol	Triazolam
Dexamethasone	Itraconazole	Nadolol	Sertraline	Verapamil

Adapted from Shiffmann [16]

Table 2.5 Sedation classification [43][a]

SEDATION

	Minimal sedation Anxiolytics	**Moderate sedation/ analgesia (Conscious Sedation)**	**Deep Sedation/ Analgesia**	**General Anesthesia**
Responsiveness	Normal response to verbal stimulation	Purposeful* to verbal or tactile Stimulation	Purposeful*response following repeated or painful stimulation	Unarousable even with painful stimulus
Airway	Unaffected	No intervention required	intervention may be required	intervention often required
Spontaneous Ventilation	Unaffected	Adequate	May be inadequate	Frequently inadequate
Cardiovascular Function	Unaffected	Usually maintained	Usually maintained	May be impared

[a]Reflex withdrawal from a painful stimulus is not considered a purposeful response

Moderate sedation/analgesia (conscious sedation) can be defined as a state where patients can give meaningful responses to verbal orders accompanied by soft tactile alerts, and a decrease in consciousness begins. Spontaneous respiration is enough and cardiovascular functions are not affected.

The patient provided with drug gives meaningful responses to painful stimuli in a state of *deep sedation/analgesia* but may not be woken up easily. The consciousness of the patient decreases more. Since the tendency to continue ventilation functions independently is reduced, support may be required for airway continuance and spontaneous respiration. Cardiovascular functions are generally protected.

Patients with unconsciousness provided by drugs under *general anesthesia* cannot be woken up even with painful stimuli. Independent continuance of ventilation functions is deteriorated; intervention is required for maintaining an open airway. If neuromuscular block constructor drug is given, positive-pressure ventilation can be required and cardiovascular functions decrease.

Surgical interventions performed with a combination of local anesthetic and sedation/analgesia in general have shorter recovery times when compared to similar interventions performed under general anesthesia or regional anesthesia [44]. Besides, sedation applied together with surgical procedures performed under local anesthesia is often preferred by both the patient and the surgeon [45]. Despite its advantages, one should be careful and cautious regarding the risks of sedation/analgesia application together with local anesthesia. In order to detect respiratory deficiencies that may arise during or after sedation, monitorization and oxygen support must be provided and the patient must be followed up [46]. Although narcotics lead to respiratory depression more than benzodiazepines, since a synergistic effect can arise during the use of sedative and narcotic drug combinations (such as midazolam + fentanyl), undesired side effects pertaining to respiration and circulation may also occur with smaller doses. Therefore, one should be more careful during their combined use [47].

Things to Remember: Box 2.15

- Sedative + narcotic drug combination yields synergistic effect.
- Side effects pertaining to respiration and circulation must be considered.
- Monitorization and oxygen support must be provided.

Benzodiazepines such as midazolam, lorazepam, and diazepam are the most commonly used agents as anxiolytic and sedative. Midazolam is a benzodiazepine with the shortest effect demonstrating sedative-hypnotic effect within 3–6 min after given intravenously. Since a deeper amnesia is provided and the recovery period is faster, its tolerance by patients is better than other benzodiazepines [48]. Lorazepam does not inhibit the cytochrome P450 CYP3A4 enzyme. Due to its characteristics, it can be preferred in liposuctions requiring high doses of lidocaine and performed with tumescent anesthesia; however, it must be kept in mind that it will extend postoperative recovery time since it has a slow effect and long elimination half-life (11–22 h) [49].

Fentanyl is a frequently preferred narcotic analgesic due to its rapid effect and effectiveness time of less than an hour. However, as stated above, since it demonstrates synergic effect with other sedative agents, it may lead to a respiration depression in even the smallest doses (25–50 μg). Narcotic analgesics such as remifentanil, alfentanil, or sufentanil have faster effects. When these agents are used, extra follow-up and monitorization are required with regard to respiration arrest. The most significant disadvantage of narcotic drugs is postoperative nausea and vomiting (PONV) [38].

Things to Remember: Box 2.16

- Midazolam is a benzodiazepine with the shortest effect.
- Lorazepam does not inhibit cytochrome P450 CYP3A4 enzyme and is appropriate for tumescent anesthesia.

Things to Remember: Box 2.17

- Propofol is a hypnotic decreasing nausea and vomiting, and its metabolism is fast.
- It must be injected slowly.

Propofol is a hypnotic agent frequently used in cosmetic procedures since it reduces postoperative nausea and vomiting [48]. It can be used on its own or in combination with many other drugs (sedative, narcotic, benzodiazepine, etc.). The fast metabolism of propofol shortens the recovery period [44]. The disadvantages of propofol use are the absence of the amnesia effect and occurrence of pain during intravenous injection. 2–3 ml 2 % lidocaine addition is enough to eliminate pain during injection. By providing oxygen and narcotic drug support, many cosmetic surgeries can be performed with a propofol and midazolam combination without any need for intubation [48]. With a midazolam addition the necessary amnestic effect is provided. Giving propofol rapidly may reduce cardiac output and thus lead to severe hypotension and respiratory depression [50].

Barbiturates such as thiopental and methohexital are also used as sedative-hypnotics. Particularly, methohexital is an alternative drug whose recovery time is fast. However, in prolonged infusions, its recovery time was recorded as longer than propofol [51].

Ketamine is an agent which has sedative-analgesic, anesthetic, and amnestic effects, does not lead to cardiovascular depression, and is derived from phencyclidine. Since its central nervous system effects constitute a case similar to catatonia, its anesthesia effect is defined as "dissociative anesthesia" [52]. Since it does not repress retching and cough reflexes, the risk for aspiration of stomach content to the lungs is significantly low [53]. When used together with benzodiazepines, any undesired postoperative psychological effects of ketamine are reduced. Table 2.6 summarizes suggested doses for certain drugs used in sedation-analgesia.

Table 2.6 Drugs and doses frequently used in sedation/analgesia

Medication	Bolus dose	Average adult dose	Continuous inf. (μ/kg/min)
Narcotic analgesics			
Fentanyl	0.3–0.7 μg/kg	25–50 μg	0.01
Alfentanil	5–7 μg/kg	30–50 μg	0.2–0.5
Remifentanil	0.5–1 μ/kg	10–25 μg	0.025–0.05
Sufentanil	0.1–0.2 μg/kg	10 μg	0.001–0.002
Morphine	0.02 mg	1–2 mg iv 5–10 mg im	–
Meperidine	0.2 mg	10–20 mg iv 50–100 mg im	–
Sedative hypnotics			
Propofol	0.2–0.5 mg/kg	10–20 mg	10–50
Midazolam	30–75 μg/kg	2.5–5 mg	0.25–0.5
Methohexital	0.2–0.5 mg/kg	10–20 mg	10–50
Diazepam	0.05–0.1 mg/kg	5–7.5 mg	–
Thiopental	0.5–1 mg/kg	25–50 mg	50–100
Dissociative anesthetic			
Ketamine	0.2–0.5 mg/kg	1020 mg	10

Adapted from Shiffmann [16]

2.5 Perioperative Considerations

It has been suggested that a 2-h period without consumption is enough for clear liquids (water, tea, coffee, pulp-free fruit juices) in elective patients. This period is 4 h for yogurt and particle-free soups and 6 h for solid food. Taking oral benzodiazepine with 150 ml water 1 h before induction for premedication purposes does not increase the gastric liquid volume [54].

Postoperative nausea and vomiting (PONV) can be observed in 80 % of patients after operation and causes trouble. Eight drugs used for preventing this condition were compared to placebos. These drugs are ondansetron, metoclopramide, droperidol, dexamethasone, tropisetron, dolasetron, granisetron, and cyclizine. In three or five of ten patients having postoperative nausea and vomiting with placebo, nausea and vomiting were prevented by the use of these drugs. Although the safety of these drugs does not differ, only two of them demonstrated 4 % side effects: sedation with droperidol and headaches with ondansetron [55]. The use of local anesthetic infusions in postoperative ache treatment provides effective pain control and leads to a decrease in PONV by decreasing the use of opioids [38]. In order to prevent PONV that may occur after the use of anesthetic agents such as nitrous oxide and narcotics, antiemetic agents can be given preoperatively [48].

Patients can be nervous before surgery. Benzodiazepines can be used in the perioperative period due to their anxiolytic and somnolence-inducing effects.

Anxiolytic drugs such as alprazolam or lorazepam can be initiated a few days before [48].

In their article published in 2008, Seruya M. et al. reported the venous thromboembolism rate as 1–2% for around 33,000 plastic surgery patients in a year. However, this rate was reported as 6.9% for venous thromboembolism and 9.4% for pulmonary emboli in patients undergoing gynecological procedures and lipectomy together with abdominoplasty. For thromboprophylaxis in high-risk patients, mechanical prophylaxis or subcutaneous heparin (low-molecular-weight heparin) or a combination of these can be used [42].

Finally, postoperative ventilation, oxygenation, and circulation values must be closely followed up. Particularly in risky patients, such as those who are obese or have OSA, hypoventilation and desaturation must be paid attention to [1].

References

1. Slabach R, Suvderhoud JP. Anesthetic considerations for abdominal wall reconstructive surgery. Emin Plast Surg. 2012;26(1):12–7.
2. ASAPS Press Center- Cosmetic Procedures in 2014. American society for aesthtetic plastic surgery Available at: http://www.surgery.org/media/statistics. Top 5 surgical procedures in 2014.
3. White PF, Smith I. Ambulatory anesthesia: past, present and future. Int Anesthesiol Clin. 1994;32(3):1–16.
4. Courtiss EH, Goldwyn RM, Joffe JM, Hannenberg AA. Anesthetic practices in ambulatory aesthetic surgery. Plast Reconstr Surg. 1994;93(4):792–801.
5. Watcha MF, White PF. Economics of anesthetic practice. Anesthesiology. 1997;86(5):1170–96.
6. Tinker JH, Dull DL, Caplan RA, Ward RJ, Cheney FW. Role of monitoring devices in prevention of anesthetic mishaps: a closed claims analysis. Anesthesiology. 1989;71(4):541–6.
7. White PF, Smith I. Impact of newer drugs and techniques on the quality of ambulatory anesthesia. J Clin Anesth. 1993;5(6 Suppl1):3S–13.
8. Natof HE. Complications associated with ambulatory surgery. JAMA. 1980;244(10):1116–8.
9. Eichhorn JH. Prevention of intraoperative anesthesia accidents and related severe injury through safety monitoring. Anesthesiology. 1989;70(4):572–7.
10. Shapiro FE, Punwani N, Rosenberg NM, Valedon A, Twersky R, Urman RD. Office-based anesthesia: safety and outcomes. Anesth Analg. 2014;119(2):276–85.
11. Keyes GR, Singer R, Iverson RE, McGuire M, Yates J, Gold A, Thompson D. Analysis of outpatient surgery center safety using an internet-based quality improvement and peer review program. Plast Reconstr Surg. 2004;113(6):1760–70.
12. Guidelines for Ambulatory Anesthesia and Surgery. Committee of origin: ambulatory surgical care (Approved by the ASA House of Delegates on 15 Oct, 2013, last amended on October 22, 2008, and reaffirmed on 16 Oct, 2013).
13. Klein JA. Tumescent technique for local anesthesia improves safety in large-volume liposuction. Plast Reconstr Surg. 1993;92(6):1085–98.
14. Guidelines for Office- Based Anesthesia. Committee of origin: ambulatory surgical care (Approved by the ASA House of Delegates on 13 Oct 1999; last amended on 21 Oct, 2009; and reaffirmed on 15 Oct, 2014).
15. A report by the american society of anesth. task force on preanesthesia evaluation. Practice advisory for preanesthesia evaluation. Anesthesiolojy. 2012;116(3).

16. Shiffmann MA, Mirrafati S editors. Anesthesia for Liposuction and Abdominoplasty. In: Aesthetic surgery of the abdominal wall. Springer science+Business Media, 2005. p 29–54.
17. Serdev N editors. Complications of liposuction. In: Advanced techniques in liposuction and fat transfer. 2011. p. 221–30.
18. ASA Physical Status Classification System. Last approved by the ASA House of Delegates on 15 Oct 2014.
19. Fleisher LA, Barash PG. Preoperative evaluation of the cardiac patient for noncardiac surgery. Yale J Biol Med. 1993;66(5):385–95.
20. Passannante AN, Tielborg M. Anesthetic management of patients with obesity and with and without sleep apnea. Clin Chest Med. 2009;30(3):569–79.
21. Flegal KM, Caroll MD, Kit BK, Ogden CL. Prevalence of obesity and trends in the distribution of body mass index among US adults, 1999–2010. JAMA. 2012;307(5):491–7.
22. Stone JG, Foex P, SWar JN, Johnson LL, Khambatta HJ, Triner L. Myocardial ischemia in untreated hypertensive patients: effect of a single small oral dose of a beta-adrenergic blocking agent. Anesthesiology. 1988;68:495–500.
23. Comfere T, Sprung J, Kumar MM, Draper M, Wilson DP, Wiiliams BA, Danielson DR, Lield L, Warner DO. Angiotensin system inhibitors in a general surgical population. Anesth Analg. 2005;100(3):636–44.
24. Hjortrup A, Sorensen C, Dyremose E, Kehlet H. Morbidity in diabetic and nondiabetic patients after abdominal surgery. Acta Chir Scand. 1985;151(5):445–7.
25. Hirsch IB, McGill JB, Cryer PE, White PF. Perioperative management of surgical patients with diabetes mellitus. Anesthesiology. 1991;74:346–59.
26. Bluman LG, Mosca L, Newman N, Simon DG. Preperative smoking habits and postoperative pulmonary complications. Chest. 1998;113(4):883–9.
27. Woods BD, Sladen RN. Perioperative considerations for the patient with asthma and bronchospasm. Br J Anaesth. 2009;103(Supl. I):i57–65.
28. Young T, Palta M, Dempsey J, Skatrud J, Weber S, Badr S. The occurrence of sleep-disordered breathing among middle -aged adults. N Engl J Med. 1993;328(17):1230–5.
29. Nugent KM, Phy M, Raj R. Obstructive sleep apnea and post-operative complications: single center data, review of literature and guidelines for practicing internists and surgeons. Surg Sci. 2012;3:65–71.
30. Liao P, Yegneswaran B, Vairavanathan S, Zilberman P, Chung F. Postoperative complications in patients with obstructive sleep apnea: a retrospective matched cohort study. Can J Anaesth. 2009;56:819–28.
31. Adams JP, Murphy PG. Obesity in anaesthesia and intensive care. Br J Anaesth. 2000;85:91–108.
32. Burns SM, Meland NB. Spinal anesthesia for abdominoplasty with liposuction: a case report. AANA J. 2007;75(2):126–8.
33. Cook TM. Combined spinal- epidural techniques. Anaesthesia. 2000;55:42–64.
34. Young MJ, Gorlin AW, Modest VE, Quraishi SA. Clinical implications of the transversus abdominis plane block in adults. Anesthesiol Res Pract. 2012;2012:731645.
35. Yu N, Long X, Lujan-Hernandez JR, Succar J, Xin X, Wang X. Transversus abdominis- plane block versus local anesthetic wound infiltraton in lower abdominal surgery: a systematic review and meta-analysis of randomized controlled trials. BMC Anesthesiol. 2014;14:121.
36. Abdallah FW, Halpern SH, Margarido CB. Transversus abdominis plane block for postoperative analgesia after Caesarean delivery performed under spinal anesthesia? A systematic review and meta-analysis. Br J Anaesth. 2012;109(5):679–87.
37. Gordley KP, Bob Basu CB. Optimal use of local anesthetics and tumescence. Semin Plast Surg. 2006;20(4):219–24.
38. Chandran GJ, Lalonde DH. A review of pain pumps in plastic surgery. Can J Plast Surg. 2010;18(1):15–8.
39. Martin AJ. pH- adjustment and discomfort caused by the intradermal injection of lignocaine. Anaesthesia. 1990;45(11):975–8.
40. Venkataram J. Tumescent liposuction: a review. J Cutan Aesthet Surg. 2008;1(2):49–57.

41. Trott SA, Beran SJ, Rohrich RJ, et al. Safety considerations and fluid resuscitation in liposuction: an analysis of 53 consecutive patients. Plast Reconstr Surg. 1998;102:2220–9.
42. Seruya M, Venturi ML, Iorio ML, Davison SP. Efficacy and safety of venous thromboembolism prophylaxis in highest risk plastic surgery patients. Plast Reconstr Surg. 2008;122(6):1701–8.
43. American Society of Anesthesiologists (ASA), Committee of Origin: Quality Management and Departmental Administration. (Approved by the ASA House of Delegates on 13 Oct 1999, and last amended on 15 Oct 2014). Continuum of Depth Sedation: Definition of General Anesthesia and Levels of Sedation/Analgesia.
44. Ghouri AF, Rmirez Ruiz MA, White PF. Effect of flumazenil on recovery after midazolam and propofol sedation. Anesthesiology. 1994;81:333–9.
45. Alishiri A, Foruzanmehr M, Mosavi SA. Comparison of sedative effect of fentanyl and remifentanyl during phacoemulsification with local anesthesia. J Anaesth. 2014;2(3):22–6.
46. Kryger ZB, Fine NA, Mustoe TA. The outcome of abdominoplasty performed under conscious sedation: Six-year experience in 153 consecutive cases. Plast Reconstr Surg. 2004;113(6):1807–17.
47. Shellay MP, Wilson P, Norman J. Sedation for fiberoptic bronchoscopy. Thorax. 1989;44(10):769–75.
48. Taub PJ, Sameer B, Hausman LM. Anesthesia for cosmetic surgery. Plast Reconstr Surg. 2010;125:1e–7.
49. Mizuno K, Katoh M, Okumura H, Nakagawa N, et al. Metabolic activation of benzodiazepines by CYP3A4. Am Soc Pharmacol Exp Ther DMD. 2009;37(2):345–51.
50. Grounds RM, Twigley AJ, Carli F, Whitwham JG, Morgan M. The haemodynamic effects of intravenous induction. Anesthesia. 1985;40:735–40.
51. Cohen M, Eisig S, Kraut RA. Comparison of recovery of propofol and methohexital sedation using an infusion pump. Am Dent Soc Anesthesiol Anesth Prog. 1996;43(1):9–13.
52. White PF, Wl W, Trevor AJ. Ketamin: its pharmacology and therapeutic uses. Anesthesiology. 1982;56:119–36.
53. Taylor PA, Ttowey RM. Depression of laryngeal reflexes during ketamin anaesthesia. Br Med J. 1971;2:688–9.
54. Ljungqvist O, Soreide E. Preoperative fasting. Br J Surg. 2003;90(4):400–6.
55. Carlisle JB, Stevenson CA. Drugs for preventing postoperative nausea and vomiting. Cochrane Database Syst Rev. 2006:19;(3):CD004125.

Chapter 3
Patient Selection

Akin Yucel

Abdominoplasty is a radical surgery that results with dramatic changes. When combined with liposuction, fat injections, and/or breast surgery, the whole torso is totally reshaped, either in single or multiple sessions. However, it is a more risky surgery with higher morbidity and mortality rates than other cosmetic procedures. Overall major complication rates after abdominoplasty is 4 %, compared with 1.4 % after other surgical cosmetic procedures [1]. Detailed preoperative evaluation, appropriate patient selection, and correct surgical planning are critical to reduce complications, improve results, and increase patient satisfaction. General health issues are important for the patient selection. A careful evaluation of the abdominal tissues, i.e., the skin, fat, and abdominal wall, is necessary for a proper technique selection and surgical strategy.

3.1 General Issues

3.1.1 Age and General Health Issues

Very old patients with general health problems are not candidates for this operation. Patients with cardiovascular problems should be consulted by cardiologist and anesthesiologist before making a decision for surgery. High blood pressure should be taken under control preoperatively. All medications that are being used should be detected and reorganized before the surgery. In healthy candidates laboratory tests

A. Yucel
Professor in Department of Plastic Reconstructive and Aesthetic Surgery,
Cerrahpaŝa Medical Faculty, Istanbul University, Istanbul, Turkey
e-mail: akinyucel@hotmail.com

K.T. Tiryaki (ed.), *Inverse Abdominoplasty*, DOI 10.1007/978-3-319-39310-0_3

are limited to complete blood count (CBC), full blood biochemistry, and standard coagulation tests. Patients with health problems need specific tests and necessary consultations (Box 3.1).

3.1.2 Respiratory Problems

Myofascial plication transiently increases intra-abdominal pressure, and patients may experience postoperative respiratory difficulties. Patients with respiratory problems should be consulted and medicated preoperatively. During surgery, myofascial plication may be abandoned, and soft tissue resection should be conservative.

3.1.3 Diabetes

Diabetes is a relative contraindication for abdominoplasty. However, if patient's general condition is good and blood glucose level is well regulated, surgery can be planned. Preoperative consultations and necessary medications should be done. In diabetic patients, a cautious surgery with less dissection, limited liposuction, and tension-free closure should be performed [2–4].

3.1.4 Clotting Problems and DVT

There is an important risk of deep vein thrombosis (DVT) and pulmonary embolism (PE) after abdominoplasty operations, and this issue should be discussed preoperatively. The risk is increased in patients who are overweight or who are using oral contraceptives. Those medications should be stopped at least 2 weeks before the surgery, if possible [5, 6]. If there is a history of previous DVT or PE or a familial tendency for hypercoagulability, a detailed laboratory analysis is necessary including factor V Leiden, as well as a hematology consultation [7] (Box 3.2).

3.1.5 Skeletal and Vertebral Problems

After abdominoplasty, a special position should be kept during first few days. This may cause severe discomfort in patients with vertebral problems and other skeletal disorders, such as disc hernia and lumbar lordosis [8]. Patients should be warned about this, and necessary precautions should be taken to minimize the discomfort.

3.1.6 Smoking

Smokers are under increased risk of ischemia, skin necrosis, fat necrosis, and wound healing problems, especially at the most distal part of the abdominal flap [3, 9]. Also intraoperative and postoperative pulmonary, cardiovascular, and cerebrovascular complications are more common in smokers [9]. Ideally, smoking should be completely stopped 6 weeks before the surgery, but practically 3 weeks of smoking-free period is sufficient. If complete cessation is not possible, surgery should either be cancelled or should be done with less dissection, limited liposuction, and closure with less tension [3].

3.1.7 Body Weight

Best cosmetic results with fewer complications can be achieved in average weight patients. Patients with a body mass index (BMI) up to 35 can be operated on, but the results would be suboptimal, and postoperative problems would be more common in overweight patients [10–12]. They should be encouraged for losing weight with diet and sports before the surgery. Patients more than 50 kg over ideal body weight should be better referred to bariatric surgery. Obesity is one of the most important reasons of morbidity and even mortality and should be considered as a relative contraindication for the procedure. However, a panniculectomy procedure can be planned in obese patients to increase life quality in terms of both weight reduction and body hygiene.

3.1.8 Pregnancy

Even though a possible pregnancy after abdominoplasty is not a contraindication, patients who consider a future pregnancy are encouraged to have the abdominoplasty be performed following the last pregnancy [13, 14].

3.1.9 Combined Procedures

Abdominoplasty is a body contouring procedure, and whole torso should be considered as a single aesthetic unit. Correcting only abdominal deformity usually results in exaggeration of other problems. Surgical planning should include breast surgery, liposuction of the abdomen, waists, and trochanteric areas, and gluteal fat injections. Those procedures can be done in the same session in suitable patients. There are several reports indicating safety of the combined procedures [15, 16]. According to Hester et al., in combined procedures, complexity of the surgical procedure is not a risk factor, but obesity is the most important risk factor increasing major complication rates [17].

Box 3.1: Relative Contraindications for Abdominoplasty

- Old patients with serious health problems
- Patients with respiratory disturbances
- Uncontrolled diabetes
- Obese patients with BMI >35 or more than 50 kg over ideal body weight
- History of hypercoagulability, DVT, and PE
- Smoking
- Patients under anticoagulant treatment
- Patients with wound healing problems, including keloid
- Vasculitis and other autoimmune diseases

Box 3.2: Preoperative Preparation for the Abdominoplasty

- Cessation of smoking at least 3 weeks prior to surgery
- Cessation of aspirin at least 3 weeks prior to surgery
- Cessation of nonsteroidal anti-inflammatory drugs (NSAIDs), vitamin E and other herbal/dietary supplements, and homeopathic products at least 1 week prior to surgery
- Encourage weight loss for the overweight patients prior to surgery
- Detailed clotting tests and/or hematology consultation for the patients with personal or family history of hypercoagulability, DVT, and PE
- Internal medicine and anesthesiology consultation for the patients with cardiovascular, respiratory, and other systemic disorders prior to surgery
- Encourage corset usage 3 weeks prior to surgery, for the patients with prominent abdominal wall laxity
- Encourage fiber-rich diet 3 days prior to surgery to avoid constipation
- Shower with a gentle antimicrobial soap on the morning of surgery

3.2 Local Issues

Establishment of the surgical strategy and selection of proper technique need a careful evaluation of the local issues such as abdominal scars, skin quality, fat depositions, and abdominal wall laxity.

Abdominal Scars Preexisting abdominal scars are of great importance in designing surgery. Traditional abdominoplasty in patients with *subcostal cholecystectomy scars* may result in deterioration of blood flow and tissue necrosis. In such patients, surgery should be done with minimal dissection and minimal tension [18]. Patients should be warned that results would be suboptimal and a tight abdomen would not be achieved after surgery.

Vertical midline scars on the contrary, usually relieve surgeons' hand, as transverse laxity can be improved by removing additional tissue transversely. The scars located in the lower abdomen, such as *appendectomy scars*, are usually removed with the specimen without any problem.

Scars from laparoscopic surgery are usually short and do not make any problem during dissection [19]. In patients with previous umbilical hernia repair, umbilical stalk might have been separated from the abdominal wall during surgery. Those patients are under risk of umbilicus necrosis after a traditional abdominoplasty. In that case, a neo-umbilicoplasty procedure should be considered. Patients should be informed about this preoperatively.

Hernias It should always be kept in mind that all scars remaining from previous abdominal surgery, including laparoscopic procedures, could be associated with unrecognized hernias. Those may not cause any difficulty in the course of flap elevation but could lead to organ injuries during liposuction [20]. Vertical midline incisions have higher risk of hernia. The risk is even higher in massive-weight-loss patients. Hernias that are not associated with an incision are most common in peri-umbilical area, especially in woman with previous pregnancies and massive-weight-loss patients. Those should be diagnosed preoperatively. For larger and complicated hernias, general surgery consultation is needed [21].

3.3 Abdominal Parameters Determining the Technique

There are five important parameters that determine the technique selection: skin quality, subcutaneous fat, intra-abdominal fat, abdominal wall laxity, and location of the umbilicus. Those should be evaluated in the preoperative examination, while the patient is standing, sitting, in supine, and flexed (diver's) positions.

3.3.1 Abdominal Skin

Skin quality, laxity, amount and location of skin excess are important for the determination of the surgical strategy. Presence of stretch marks is a sign of bad skin quality. In young, nulliparous patients with good skin quality, liposuction alone may be enough to solve the problems.

Skin laxity is tested while the patient is in supine position. If the abdominal skin could be pulled down easily, this means the patient is a good candidate for a full abdominoplasty. Patients with firm skin should be considered for liposuction and/or mini-abdominoplasty procedures.

The amount of skin excess should also be evaluated. If there is skin excess both above and below umbilicus, patient should be considered for a full abdominoplasty. If the skin excess is only under the umbilicus, a mini-abdominoplasty or a floating umbilicus technique would be more suitable. This type of patients usually has a high-located umbilicus.

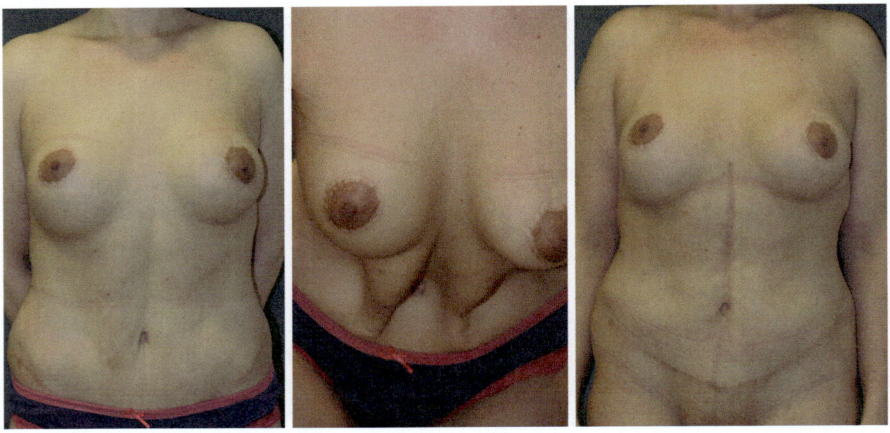

Fig. 3.1 View of the abdomen of a massive-weight-loss patient in diver's position after belt lipectomy. Vertical skin excess has been removed; however, horizontal skin excess still persists. A fleur-de-lys procedure was performed afterwards

Classical abdominoplasty techniques usually treat only the vertical skin excess. However, especially in massive-weight-loss patients, there is also horizontal skin excess. This can best be best determined when the patient is in diver's position, i.e., flexed forward. If there is significant horizontal skin excess, a fleur-de-lys procedure with vertical midline incision should be considered [22]. The remaining scars should be discussed with the patients preoperatively. If decision is not clear, vertical excision could be done as a secondary procedure after initial abdominoplasty (Fig. 3.1).

The amount of vertical skin excess also determines the length of the incision. Lateral skin excess can be removed by high lateral tension abdominoplasty [23]. However, if the skin excess is circumferential, especially in massive-weight-loss patients, a belt lipectomy procedure should be considered [24].

3.3.2 Subcutaneous Fat

The amount and location of the subcutaneous fat should be examined carefully. In lipoabdominoplasty procedures, liposuction is a part of the operation. Wide liposuction allows easy mobilization of the abdominal skin without undermining, and contrary to the common belief, it is a safe procedure in terms of blood circulation [25]. The areas to be suctioned should be determined and marked preoperatively. In body sculpting procedures, whole abdomen, pubic area, flanks, back, and trochanteric areas are suctioned prior to abdominoplasty. Also fat injections to the gluteal area and supratrochanteric depressions should be considered, if necessary. Ultrasonic techniques, such as VASER, are getting more popular in abdominal shaping. Hi-def liposuction with VASER allows surgeon to create anatomical details such as six-pack abs [26]. Precise liposhaping should be considered only in patients with ideal weight and sporting regularly.

Patients with good skin quality and skin excess can be treated with liposuction alone. Hi-def procedures can also be considered in selected patients. However, it

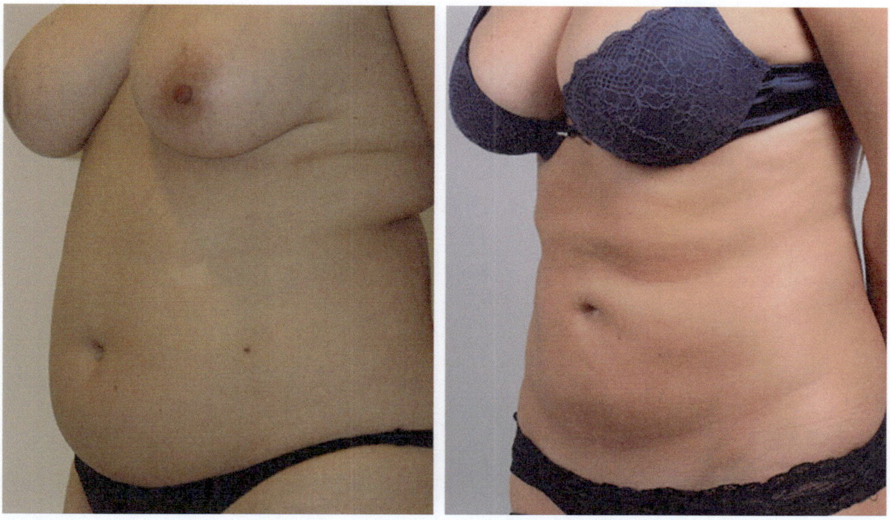

Fig. 3.2 It should be remembered that even in young, nulliparous patients with good skin quality, excessive liposuction might result in skin irregularities

should always be kept in mind that excessive liposuction, even in young patients with tight skin, may result in irregularities especially in the hypogastric area and skin accumulation just over the umbilicus (Fig. 3.2).

3.3.3 Intra-abdominal Fat

Visceral fat accumulation occurs with age and is more likely to be found in men. Women also accumulate this type of fat as they approach menopause. Alcohol consumption also increases visceral fat accumulation. These patients usually have a distended abdomen with a little subcutaneous fat. The presence of substantial visceral fat accumulation prevents any successful result even if extensive muscular tightening would be performed (Fig. 3.3). It should be kept in mind that patients with excessive intraperitoneal fat cannot be treated by any abdominal contour procedure [27]. Such patients are contraindicated for any abdominal surgery may it be liposuction or abdominoplasty. These patients are directed to dieticians or bariatric surgery centers. It should also be remembered that patients with that body type are under more risk of cardiac problems [28].

3.3.4 Abdominal Wall

Musculofascial laxity is common in patients with multiple pregnancies or after massive weight loss. In majority of male patients, abdominal wall laxity is not present and there is no need for myofascial tightening [29]. Abdominal wall laxity is best

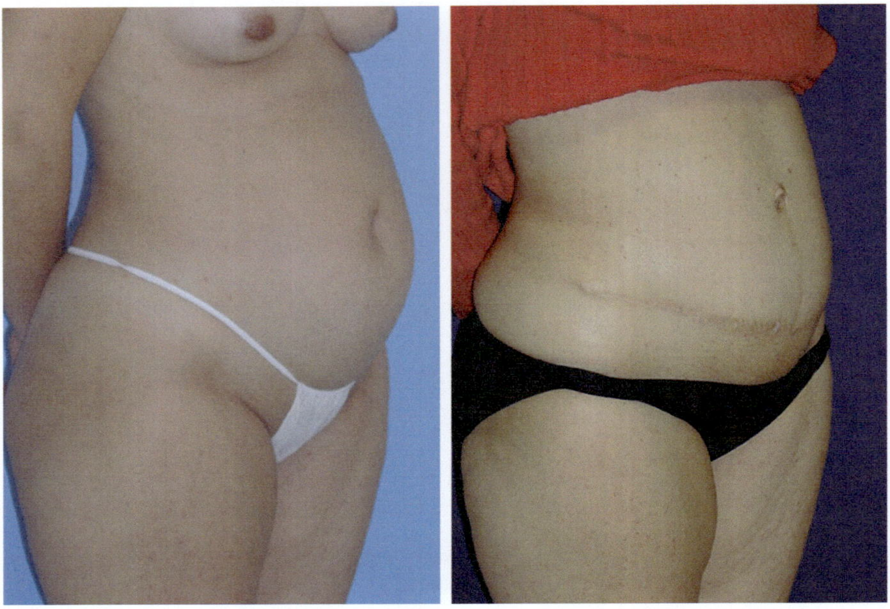

Fig. 3.3 Patient with significant intra-abdominal fat accumulation and lumbar lordosis. Although a full abdominoplasty was performed, there is no improvement except for adding an ugly scar

determined while the patient is wanted to do crunches in supine position. Ventral and periumbilical hernias can also be examined in the same way. A thick subcutaneous fat layer may obscure the hernia, and careful examination should be performed [20, 21]. In patients with visceral fattening, even in presence of abdominal wall laxity, operation should be postponed after weight loss.

As indicated previously in the chapter, myofascial tightening may cause respiratory disturbances and should be done either conservatively or cancelled in patients with respiratory problems [27].

3.3.5 Position of the Umbilicus

Patients with high-seated umbilicus do not have enough excess skin to allow traditional abdominoplasty without a high transverse or vertical midline scar. If there is no skin excess above the umbilicus, a mini-abdominoplasty procedure combined with liposuction could be good solution. If there is skin excess above the umbilicus with myofascial laxity, floating umbilicus technique with low placement of a full transverse abdominal scar, abdominal flap undermining, more inferior umbilical repositioning, flank liposuction, and plication of diastasis recti from xiphoid to pubis should be considered [30]. If the skin excess is not present, endoscopic myofascial repair and inferior repositioning of the umbilicus may be a better solution [31] (Fig. 3.4)

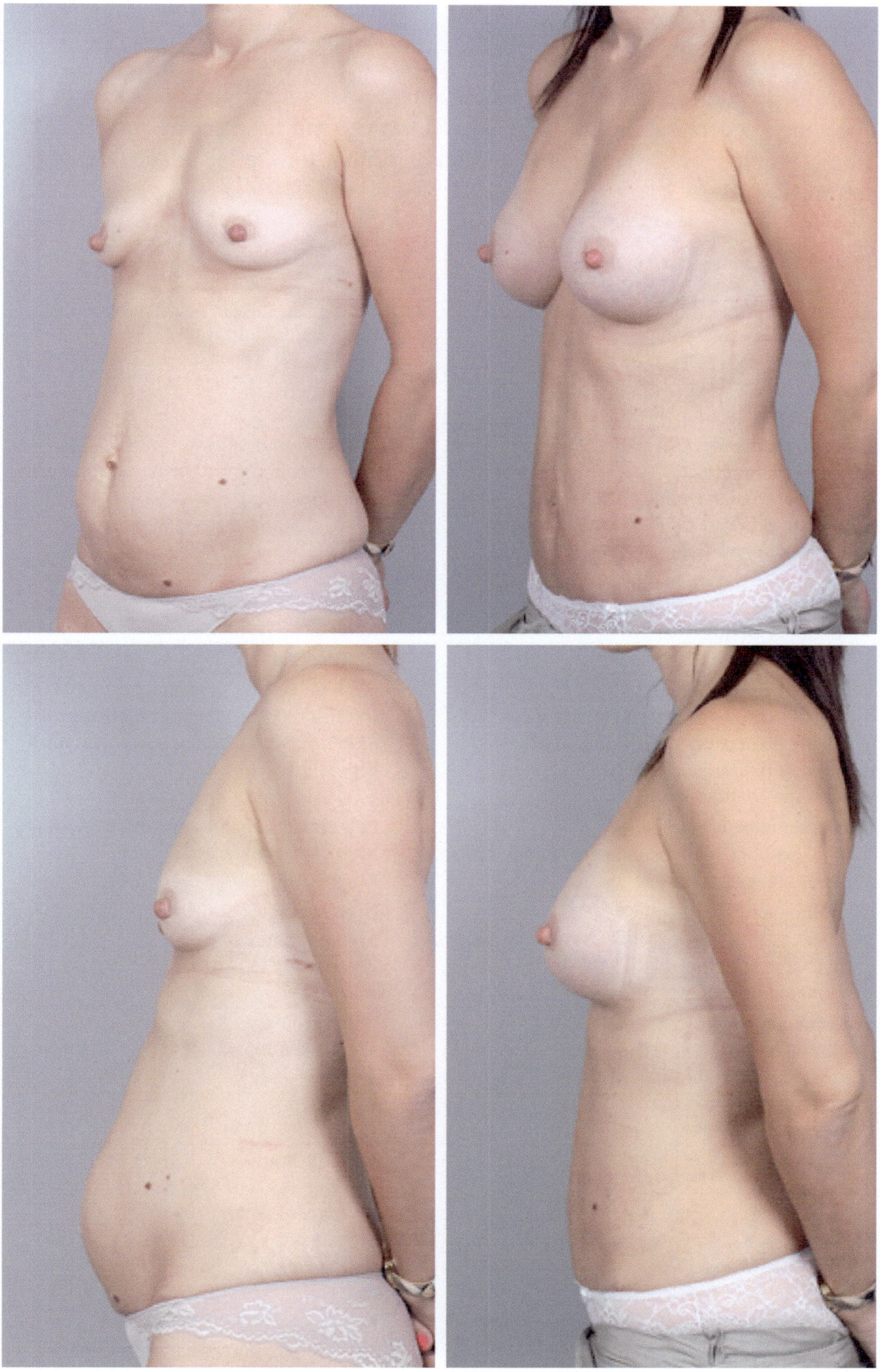

Fig. 3.4 Floating umbilicus procedure with myofascial repair, inferior repositioning of the umbilicus, skin resection from the lower abdomen, combined with breast augmentation (14 months postoperatively)

3.4 Technique Selection

There is a wide spectrum of surgical techniques varying from liposuction to belt lipectomy, depending on the abdominal deformity and tissue characteristics [32]. Surgical strategies are summarized as an algorithm for the technique selection is presented in Table 3.1:

Table 3.1 Technique selection

Patient and tissue characteristics	Technique
Young, nulliparous patient Good skin quality No skin excess No abdominal wall laxity	Liposuction only
Good to moderate skin quality High-seated umbilicus No skin excess above the umbilicus Moderate skin excess below the umbilicus No abdominal wall laxity	Mini-abdominoplasty Skin resection from the lower abdomen Liposuction (±)
Good to moderate skin quality No skin excess Abdominal wall laxity (+)	Endoscopic abdominoplasty Myofascial repair No skin excision Liposuction (±)
Good to moderate skin quality Minimal skin excess above the umbilicus Moderate skin excess below the umbilicus High-seated umbilicus Abdominal wall laxity (+)	Floating umbilicus technique Inferior repositioning of umbilicus Skin resection from the lower abdomen Liposuction (±)
Moderate to bad skin quality Skin excess both above and below the umbilicus Abdominal wall laxity (+)	Full abdominoplasty/lipoabdominoplasty Myofascial repair Liposuction (±)
Bad skin quality Skin excess both above and below the umbilicus Skin excess laterally Abdominal wall laxity (+)	High lateral tension abdominoplasty Myofascial repair Liposuction (±)
Massive-weight-loss patient Bad skin quality Skin excess both above and below the umbilicus Circumferential skin excess Abdominal wall laxity (+)	Belt lipectomy Myofascial repair Liposuction (±)
Massive-weight-loss patient Bad skin quality Skin excess both above and below the umbilicus Circumferential skin excess Horizontal skin excess Abdominal wall laxity (+)	Belt lipectomy Fleur-de-lys-type skin resection Myofascial repair Liposuction (±)
Excessive intra-abdominal fat accumulation	No surgery Refer to dietitian or bariatric surgery
Obese patients with BMI >35 Patients with more than 50 kg over ideal weight	Refer to dietitian or bariatric surgery Panniculectomy from the lower abdomen, if necessary

1. *Liposuction only:* In young patients with good skin quality, liposuction alone may improve abdominal appearance. However, it should be done conservatively because even in young patients, there is always a risk of irregularities as emphasized previously.
2. *Mini-abdominoplasty:* Patients with high-seated umbilicus are not suitable for a full abdominoplasty. In patients with skin excess below the umbilicus, wide liposuction combined with skin resection from the lower abdomen is a good solution (Fig. 3.5). If myofascial laxity is present, floating umbilicus technique with myofascial repair and inferior repositioning of the umbilicus might be the appropriate technique.
3. *Endoscopic abdominoplasty:* Patients with significant abdominal wall laxity, but no skin excess, are good candidates for endoscopic myofascial repair, combined with liposuction and/or skin excision from the lower abdomen.
4. *Full abdominoplasty:* Patients with skin laxity both above and below the umbilicus are candidates for full abdominoplasty procedure. Myofascial tightening is also performed in majority of patients (Fig. 3.6). Amount of skin excision depends on the type of skin laxity, varying from high lateral tension abdominoplasty to belt lipectomy combined with fleur-de-lys-type skin resection.

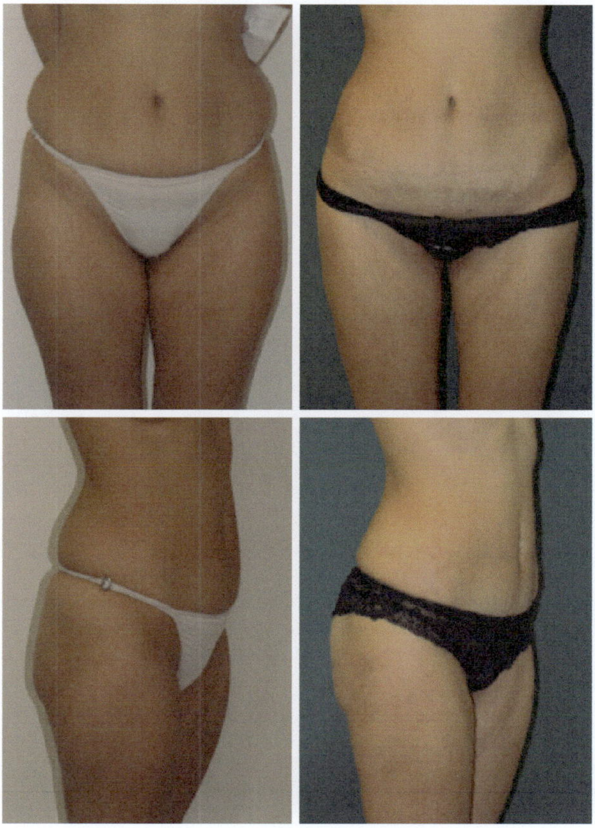

Fig. 3.5 A mini-abdominoplasty procedure with wide liposuction, gluteal fat injections, and skin resection from the lower abdomen (22 months postoperatively)

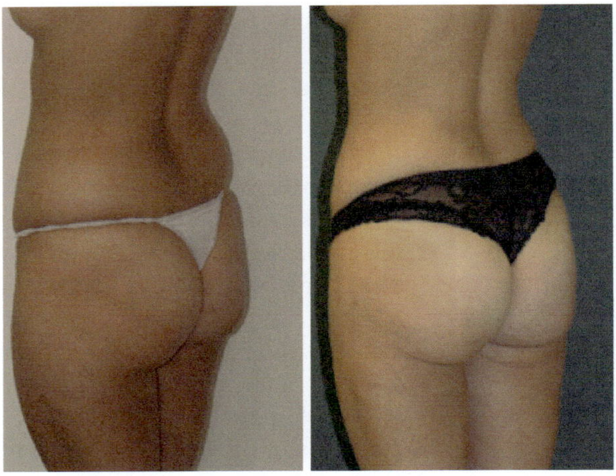

Fig. 3.5 (continued)

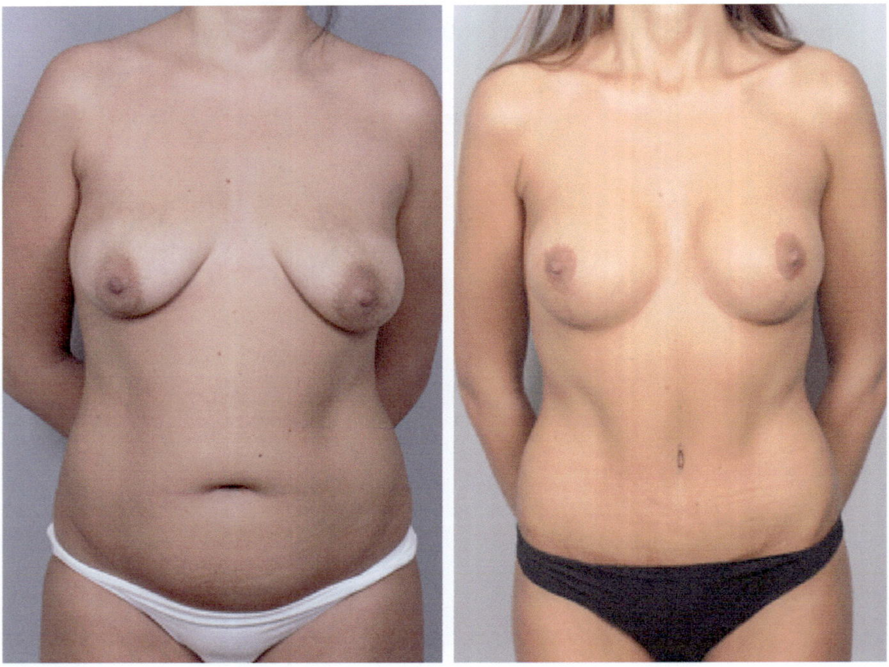

Fig. 3.6 In suitable patients, combined procedures give successful results. Pre- and postoperative views after full lipoabdominoplasty with myofascial repair, wide liposuction and fat injections, and augmentation mastopexy (21 months postoperatively)

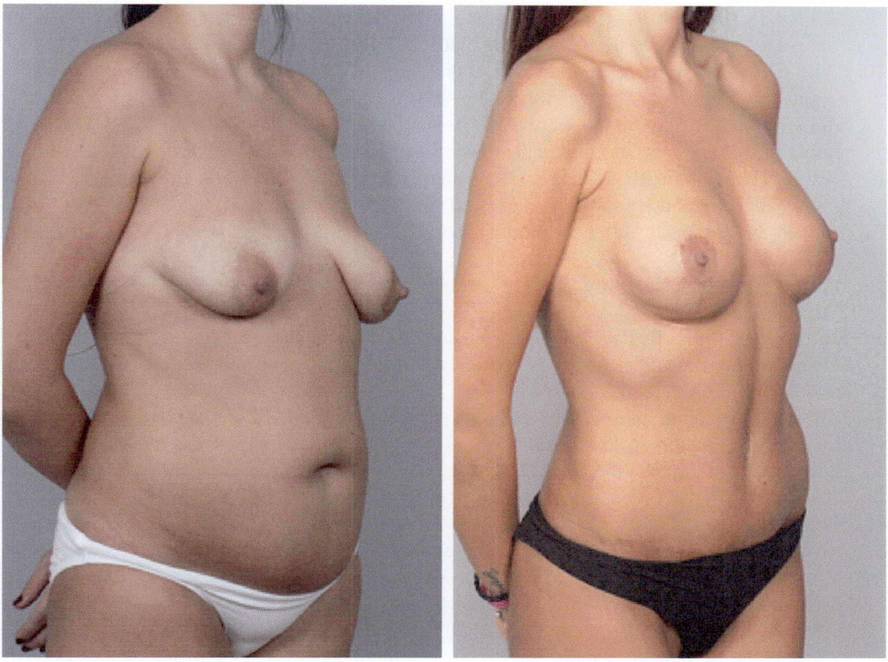

Fig. 3.6 (continued)

References

1. Winocour J, Gupta V, Ramirez JR, Shack RB, Grotting JC, Higdon KK. Abdominoplasty: risk factors, complication rates, and safety of combined procedures. Plast Reconstr Surg. 2015;136(5):597–606.
2. Guyuron B, Raszewski R. Undetected diabetes and the plastic surgeon. Plast Reconstr Surg. 1990;86(3):471–4.
3. Manassa EH, Hertl CH, Olbrisch RR. Wound healing problems in smokers and nonsmokers after 132 abdominoplasties. Plast Reconstr Surg. 2003;111(6):2082–7. discussion 2088–9.
4. Hensel JM, Lehman Jr JA, Tantri MP, Parker MG, Wagner DS, Topham NS. An outcomes analysis and satisfaction survey of 199 consecutive abdominoplasties. Ann Plast Surg. 2001;46(4):357–63.
5. Blickstein D, Blickstein I. Oral contraception and thrombophilia. Curr Opin Obstet Gynecol. 2007;19(4):370–6.
6. Van Vlijmen EF, Brouwer JL, Veeger NJ, Eskes TK, de Graeff PA, van der Meer J. Oral contraceptives and the absolute risk of venous thromboembolism in women with single or multiple thrombophilic defects: results from a retrospective family cohort study. Arch Intern Med. 2007;167(3):282–9.
7. Friedman T, O'Brien Coon D, Michaels VJ, Bontempo F, Young VL, Clavijo JA, Rubin JP. Hereditary coagulopathies: practical diagnosis and management for the plastic surgeon. Plast Reconstr Surg. 2010;125(5):1544–52.
8. Matarasso A, Matarasso DM, Matarasso EJ. Abdominoplasty: classic principles and technique. Clin Plast Surg. 2014;41(4):655–72.

9. Krueger JK, Rohrich RJ. Clearing the smoke: the scientific rationale for tobacco abstention with plastic surgery. Plast Reconstr Surg. 2001;108(4):1063–73. discussion 1074–7.
10. Swift RW, Matarasso A, Rankin M. Abdominoplasty and abdominal contour surgery: a national plastic surgery survey. Plast Reconstr Surg. 2007;119(1):426–7.
11. Kim J, Stevenson TR. Abdominoplasty, liposuction of the flanks, and obesity: analyzing risk factors for seroma formation. Plast Reconstr Surg. 2006;117(3):773–9. discussion 780–1.
12. Vastine VL, Morgan RF, Williams GS, Gampper TJ, Drake DB, Knox LK, Lin KY. Wound complications of abdominoplasty in obese patients. Ann Plast Surg. 1999;42(1):34–9.
13. Wallach SG. Pregnancy after abdominoplasty. Plast Reconstr Surg. 2002;110(7):1805. author reply 1805–6.
14. Borman H. Pregnancy in the early period after abdominoplasty. Plast Reconstr Surg. 2002;109(1):396–7.
15. Stevens WG, Repta R, Pacella SJ, Tenenbaum MJ, Cohen R, Vath SD, Stoker DA. Safe and consistent outcomes of successfully combining breast surgery and abdominoplasty: an update. Aesthet Surg J. 2009;29(2):129–34.
16. Dillerud E. Abdominoplasty combined with suction lipoplasty: a study of complications, revisions, and risk factors in 487 cases. Ann Plast Surg. 1990;25(5):333–8. discussion 339–43.
17. Hester Jr TR, Baird W, Bostwick 3rd J, Nahai F, Cukic J. Abdominoplasty combined with other major surgical procedures: safe or sorry? Plast Reconstr Surg. 1989;83(6):997–1004.
18. Karthikesalingam A, Kitcat M, Malata CM. Abdominoplasty in patients with and without pre-existing scars: a retrospective comparison. J Plast Reconstr Aesthet Surg. 2011;64(3):369–74.
19. El-Khatib HA, Bener A. Abdominal dermolipectomy in an abdomen with pre-existing scars: a different concept. Plast Reconstr Surg. 2004;114(4):992–7.
20. Zakine G, Baruch J, Dardour JC, Flageul G. Perforation of viscera, a dramatic complication of liposuction: a review of 19 cases evaluated by experts in France between 2000 and 2012. Plast Reconstr Surg. 2015;135(3):743–50.
21. Neinstein RM, Matarasso A, Abramson DL. Concomitant abdominoplasty and umbilical hernia repair using the Ventralex hernia patch. Plast Reconstr Surg. 2015;135(4):1021–5.
22. Duff CG, Aslam S, Griffiths RW. Fleur-de-Lys abdominoplasty—a consecutive case series. Br J Plast Surg. 2003;56(6):557–66.
23. Lockwood TE. Maximizing aesthetics in lateral-tension abdominoplasty and body lifts. Clin Plast Surg. 2004;31(4):523–37.
24. Aly A, Mueller M. Circumferential truncal contouring: the belt lipectomy. Clin Plast Surg. 2014;41(4):765–74.
25. Saldanha OR, Azevedo SF, Delboni PS, Saldanha Filho OR, Saldanha CB, Uribe LH. Lipoabdominoplasty: the Saldanha technique. Clin Plast Surg. 2010;37(3):469–81.
26. Hoyos AE, Millard JA. VASER-assisted high-definition liposculpture. Aesthet Surg J. 2007;27(6):594–604.
27. Graça Neto L, Araújo LR, Rudy MR, Auersvald LA, Graf R. Intraabdominal pressure in abdominoplasty patients. Aesthetic Plast Surg. 2006;30(6):655–8.
28. Barry DR, Utzschneider KM, Tong J, Gaba K, Leotta DF, Brunzell JD, Easterling TR. Intraabdominal fat, insulin sensitivity, and cardiovascular risk factors in postpartum women with a history of preeclampsia. Am J Obstet Gynecol. 2015;213(1):104.
29. Matarasso A. The male abdominoplasty. Clin Plast Surg. 2004;31(4):555–69.
30. Colwell AS, Kpodzo D, Gallico 3rd GG. Low scar abdominoplasty with inferior positioning of the umbilicus. Ann Plast Surg. 2010;64(5):639–44.
31. Eaves 3rd FF, Nahai F, Bostwick 3rd J. Endoscopic abdominoplasty and endoscopically assisted miniabdominoplasty. Clin Plast Surg. 1996;23(4):599–616. discussion 617.
32. Saltz R. Two position comprehensive approach to abdominoplasty. Clin Plast Surg. 2014;41(4):681–704.

Chapter 4
The Theory of Inverse Abdominoplasty

Tunc Tiryaki

4.1 Introduction

What would be an ideal abdominoplasty technique?

- First of all, this technique shall be fast and at the same time safe.
- Second, it shall have a simple design with a reproducible result under all circumstances. It shall be painless!
- Third, the result shall be predictable so that neither the surgeon nor the patient do not need to worry about surprises like an unwanted T-scar.
- Lastly, the aesthetic outcome shall resemble the archetypal beauty of the abdomen with lateral grooves, rectus folds, and linea alba.

Even though the abdominoplasty procedure is one of the oldest procedures of our field, it would be a wishful thinking that all these criteria are fulfilled by the conventional approach.

In this chapter, we are going to first of all analyze the beauty concepts of the abdominal area we are trying to achieve. Then, we will focus on the functional anatomy of the region as well as the forces we need to manipulate in order to shape the abdomen to obtain the desired outcome. The inverse approach described here is meant to fulfill all the criteria above. It will ease the procedure immensely, shorten the dissection time and length, reduce the duration of the procedure, and dismiss the need of a possible vertical scar for skin closure. Most importantly, an aesthetically supreme waist definition, a more muscly appearance due to false rectus folds, and a better reverse lifting of the groin are obtained.

Inverse abdominoplasty is not an aversion or a type of reverse abdominoplasty, where the incision is just below the inframammary fold and the abdominal skin flap is elevated and pulled upward [1, 2]. In inverse approach, like in a traditional

T. Tiryaki
Department of Plastic Surgery, Cellest Plastic Surgery Center, Istanbul, Turkey
e-mail: drtunctiryaki@gmail.com

K.T. Tiryaki (ed.), *Inverse Abdominoplasty*, DOI 10.1007/978-3-319-39310-0_4

abdominoplasty procedure, the lower abdominal skin is elevated, the flap superior to the umbilicus is pulled downward, and the skin excess lower to the navel is excised [3]. In this technique, however, the surgery doesn't start with a cesarian section level incision low over the mons pubis but with a *seagull shape supra-umbilical incision*. After this initial midline incision, the flap superior to the umbilicus is elevated first; after the umbilicus is separated, the flap inferior to it is dissected toward the mons pubis. Whatever the technique used, the basic goals of surgery are the removal of the excess loose skin and tightening the underlying musculofascial system employing the least conspicuous incision [4].

Acquired abdominal contour deformities can be the result of circumstances like weight gain or fluctuations, pregnancy, hormones, medications, lifestyle, previous surgical incisions, or simply aging. Pregnancy as the most common example induces irreversible changes in the vertebral column, ribs, pelvis, and most importantly in the tone of the musculoaponeurotic system [5]. Post-bariatric patients can get rid of the excess subcutaneous fat volume but usually end up with loose, draping skin. In addition, operations on the abdominal wall and hernias may further weaken and partially denervate the musculoaponeurotic system [6]. Exercise and weight loss can improve the abdominal contour up to a degree but certain groups of people cannot reach their desired goals.

In any case, the resulting deformity is a combination of a three-dimensional expansion of the abdominal cavity and skin excess in horizontal as well as in a vertical plane. A conventional full abdominoplasty is the most commonly performed method to try to address all the problems mentioned at once.

Unfortunately, this procedure is usually associated not only with long operation times but also a painful recovery period, highly located suprapubic scars, and significant complication rates like seroma and necrosis. In borderline cases as well as reoperative abdominoplasty patients, starting the operation from the inferior incision would mean to burn the bridges from the start of the procedure and may result in unwanted or unplanned T-scars. Using the inferior incision as the starting point of the procedure would necessitate the undermining of a long superior flap, which is one of the main reasons of long operative time and difficulty. Another issue is the aesthetic outcome, which cannot be reduced to a simple excision of the skin excess and primary closure of the defect. The aesthetic results of conventional abdominoplasty do not necessarily mimic the eminences and grooves of the archetype of a beautiful tummy. Postoperative pain is also an important factor decreasing the number of the abdominoplasty candidates.

In contrast to conventional abdominoplasty with an inferior start incision, an inverse abdominoplasty with *a supra-umbilical midline start* facilitates the surgeon to perform the procedure in much shorter time due to shorter flaps superiorly and inferiorly. Also, there is never a need for a T-scar at the closure. This approach, using maneuvers like *seagull shape dermolipectomy*, *horizontal-vertical plication* of the rectus sheath for three-dimensional musculoaponeurotic tightening, and *umbilical anchorage,* using the fascia as an anchor for the umbilical stalk as well as the midline of the skin flap, would be extremely effective to address the problems referred before as well as to create an aesthetically superior outcome.

Points to Remember

- Starting with an inferior incision and undermining of the long superior flap is the main reason of the long operative time and difficulty.
- In borderline cases and reoperative abdominoplasty patients, an initial inferior incision would burn the bridges from the start and may result in unwanted and unplanned T-scars.
- Postoperative pain is a major issue decreasing the number of the abdominoplasty candidates, which shall be dealt with.
- Conventional abdominoplasty with a simple abdominal tuck will not create satisfactory aesthetic outcomes, mimicking the archetypal beauty of the abdomen.

4.2 Patient Selection

The classification of the abdominal deformity is the keystone for choosing the appropriate surgical technique, which can be liposuction, endoscopic abdominoplasty, mini abdominoplasty, or full abdominoplasty [7].

The three parameters help us to decide about the necessary procedure:

(a) *The visceral fat accumulation*
(b) *The skin quality*
(c) *The abdominal wall laxity*

We evaluate these parameters in the preoperative examination, which is performed in the standing, sitting, and flexed (diver's) positions, and body proportions, musculoskeletal architecture, umbilical variations, hernias, and scars are noted [8] (Table 4.1). The skin quality, degree of subcutaneous/visceral fat accumulation, and extent of muscular diastasis or weakness are discussed with the patient in front of a mirror. As shown on the chart and table, the crucial parameter in decision-making process is the skin quality as well as stretch marks and skin excess.

Class V: The presence of substantial visceral fat accumulation prevents any successful result even if extensive muscular tightening would be performed. Such patients are contraindicated for any abdominal surgery may it be liposuction or abdominoplasty and are directed to dieticians or bariatric surgery centers (Table 4.2).

Class I: On the contrary to visceral fat accumulation, subcutaneous fat accumulation can be solved with liposuction only if the skin elasticity is good without any stretch marks/striae and good abdominal wall integrity.

Class II: If skin quality is good but existing wall laxity is prominent, an endoscopic abdominoplasty together with or without liposuction or mini abdominoplasty might be chosen.

Class III: Medium level skin laxity, particularly with short upper abdomen, and the resulting lack of enough postsurgical skin cover may necessitate a combination of mini abdominoplasty with or without floating umbilicus and upper abdominal plication. It is to be noted that performing mini abdominoplasty without abdominal plication is a sure way to patient dissatisfaction. This is valid particularly for an incomplete plication covering only the lower part of the abdomen. In such cases, the tightening of the lower abdomen will result in bulging of the upper abdomen.

Class IV: If both wall integrity and skin elasticity are poor, a full inverse abdominoplasty should be considered.

As a summary, the typical patient for standard abdominoplasty has excessive, loose, sagging, abdominal skin, lax abdominal fascial wall, and/or diastasis recti with minimum visceral fat accumulation [9].

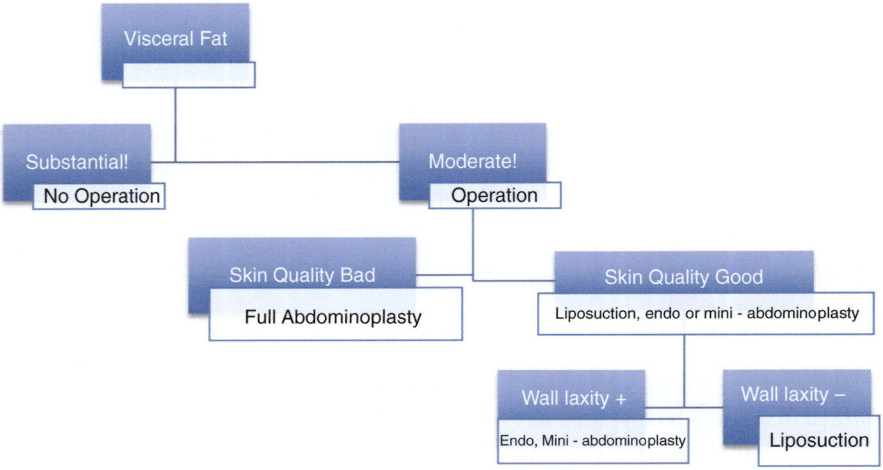

Table 4.1 In the decision-making process, the first parameter shall be the amount of visceral fat. If there is a substantial amount of abdominal visceral fat, any surgery would result in suboptimal outcomes, so the patient shall be encouraged to lose weight first. With a moderate amount of visceral fat, the decisive factor will be the skin quality. Bad skin quality with striae is a clear indication for abdominoplasty, whereas patients with good skin quality might benefit greatly from a liposuction or endoscopic abdominoplasty depending on the abdominal wall laxity

Table 4.2 Classification of abdominoplasty candidates

Class	Visceral fat	Skin elasticity	Musculofascial tonus	Treatment
Class I	–+	Good	Good	Liposuction
Class II	–+	Good	Moderate	Endoscopic abdominoplasty
Class III	–+	Average	Moderate	Mini abdominoplasty
Class IV	–+	Poor	[a]	Inverse abdominoplasty
Class V	++	[a]	[a]	No surgery

[a]Insignificant

Things to Remember:

- Three parameters: *the visceral fat accumulation, the skin quality, and the abdominal wall laxity* help us to decide about the necessary procedure.
- The presence of substantial visceral fat accumulation prevents any successful result even if extensive muscular tightening would be performed.
- Moderate visceral fat accumulation cannot be treated without abdominal wall plication.
- Subcutaneous fat accumulation with a good skin quality and elasticity can be solved only with liposuction.
- Medium level skin laxity, particularly with short upper abdomen, may necessitate a combination of mini abdominoplasty and upper abdominal plication.
- Performing mini abdominoplasty without abdominal plication or with incomplete plication for the lower abdomen will result in even worse outcomes with rebound bulging of the upper belly.

4.3 Anatomy of a Beautiful Belly

Even a cursory perusal of the imagery depicting the ideal stomach in the popular culture – advertising, films, television, non-medical literature and so on – is required to appreciate that there is a dominant perception of what the abdomen, especially the female abdomen, should look like: flat and tight without overly obvious fat deposits. Women frequently desire to have an "hourglass" or "coke bottle" shape formed by the relative thinness of waist and abdomen relative to the fuller bustline and hips. Men often search for a "V-shape" with a waist area smaller than the shoulders and without full hips, and ones aspiring to an implied athleticism may seek a "six pack," in which the individual muscles of the frontal abdomen stand out in relief.

Although this last effect is perhaps best achieved through long exercise, medical science does have its methods. Aside from our brief nod to common beauty standards, medical and scholarly literature and experience confirm that most people seeking the help of medical professionals for problems related to self-image in this area of the body much prefer to conform to these exact same cultural beauty norms; abdominal aesthetic intervention usually tries to replicate this archetypal shape in order to be considered successful. So the question for doctors is: How are these precise curves sculpted?

Abdominoplasty, liposuction, and other related procedures have been extensively researched and highly effective techniques have been developed. A surgeon looking to perform these operations has an abundance of resources to turn to for aid. However, one fact that can never change is that successful abdominal aesthetic intervention requires a detailed, three-dimensional familiarity with the anatomy of the body's midsection.

There are distinct abdominal surface landmarks, dependent upon subdermal features, which define the shape of an attractive abdomen. Much of abdominoplasty involves resituating these visible lines and masses relative to one another.

The abdomen (less formally called the *belly, stomach, tummy*) constitutes the part of the body between the thorax (chest) and pelvis. Midway across horizontally, a slight furrow extends from the ensiform cartilage (also known as the xiphoid process) above to the pubic symphysis, constituting the *linea alba* in the abdominal wall. It is so called because it is made mostly of connective tissue (linea alba being Latin for "white line"). Since it is made up mostly of collagen and contains no primary blood vessels or nerves, it is a favored path for incisions. At about its vertical midpoint lies the bellybutton, better known as the umbilicus or navel.

On either side of the "white line," broad recti muscles (sometimes, and not unambiguously correctly, known simply as the *abs*) stand out in muscular people. The outline of these muscles is interrupted by three or more transverse depressions indicating the *linea transversae*, or sometimes the tendinous intersections. These allow us forward flexion, as when we bend over to pick something up or do sit-up exercises. There is usually one near the ensiform cartilage, one at the umbilicus, and one between. Occasionally, in people with very low body fat, a fourth is visible below the umbilicus. It is the combination of the linea alba and the linea transversae which form the abdominal "six-pack" sought after by many fitness junkies and male models.

The *linea semilunaris* (also semilunar line or Spigelian line) is a curved tendinous line found on either side of the rectus abdominis muscle. Each corresponds with the lateral border of the rectus abdominis, extends from the cartilage of the ninth rib to the pubic tubercle.

The upper lateral limit of the abdomen is the *costal margin* (at or near the *subcostal plane*) formed by the cartilages of the false ribs [8–10] joining one another. The lower lateral limit is the anterior crest of the ilium, which runs from the anterior superior spine of the ilium to the spine of the pubis. These lower limits are marked by visible grooves [10]. These lines are demarking the grooves and eminences of the abdominal area. The hourglass appearance is the result of the concavity of the core muscles, the external oblique, the internal oblique, and the transverse abdominis between the thorax and the hips.

Ideally, there is a median tissue prominence marking the rectus muscles between the costal margin and the pubis, which is vertically divided by linea alba. This prominence has two grooves on both sides, which are delineated by the linea semilunaris (Fig. 4.1a).

4.4 Manipulating the Forces Effecting the Abdominal Shape

In order to mimic this ideal anatomy and to create a beautiful abdominoplasty result, we should fulfill the following basic aesthetic goals:

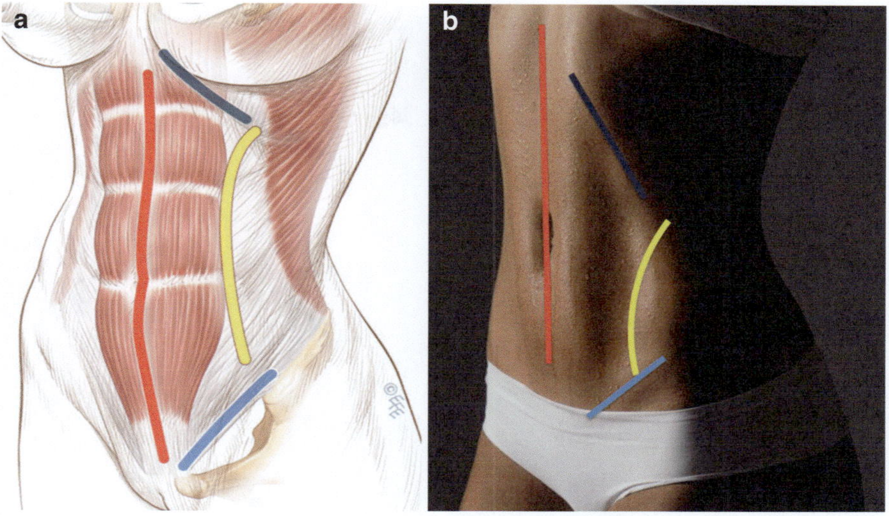

Fig. 4.1 (**a**, **b**) (*left*) Anatomy of the human abdomen and a modern example of a human female abdomen with superficial landmarks: linea alba, linea semilunaris, Poupart's ligament, costal margin

1. **Coke bottle shape with bilateral grooves**: We have to re-create the coke bottle shape by enforcing the concavity of the core muscles of the abdomen. The bilateral hollowing, following the *linea semilunaris,* which corresponds to the lateral border of the rectus abdominis, extending from the cartilage of the ninth rib to the pubic tubercle, is to be shaped (Fig. 4.2).
2. **Rectus muscle eminence**: A median tissue prominence between the costal margin and the pubis is to be recreated to fashion the rectus muscle folds illusion.
3. **Recreating linea alba**: A new midline rift, corresponding with the existing linea alba, should vertically divide the mentioned tissue eminence (Fig. 4.1b).

In order to get the mentioned bottleneck appearance, the bilateral grooves, and the rectus muscle eminence with the midline rift, we need to fashion two lateral grooves: a median tissue prominence and a line dividing this tissue into twofold during the surgery. Let's take step-by-step look at the surgical maneuvers used in order to achieve these anatomical landmarks.

1. **The coke bottle shape and lateral grooves** are fashioned by the contribution of the following surgical maneuvers:

   A. **Inverse seagull incision**: The inverse start with the superior bilaterally upward curving incision enables the surgeon to design a relative paramedian skin gap and median skin excess. This is the first step to create a median skin excess as well as the medial pull of the waist (Fig. 4.3a, *black arrow*).

   B. **Tunnel dissection**: Upper flap elevation is done with minimal superolateral dissection. This will ensure the safety of the vascular supply for the flap, but more importantly it will keep the attachments between the superior flap and

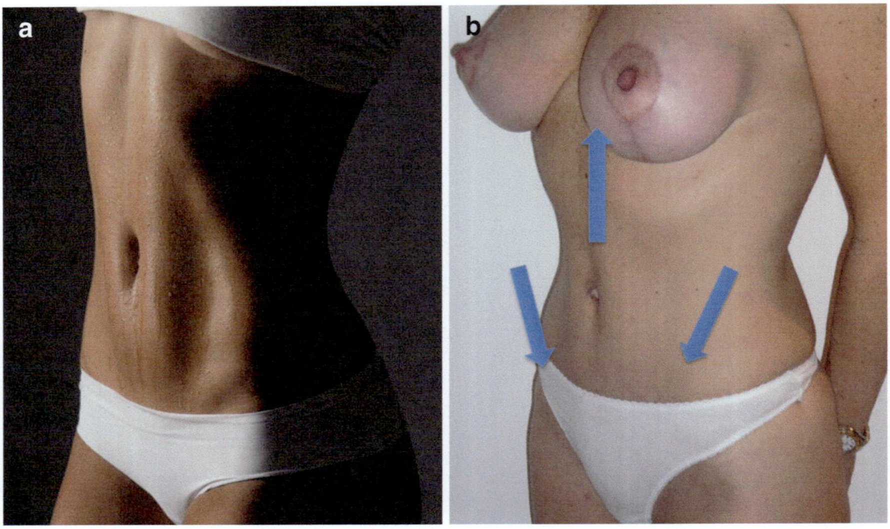

Fig. 4.2 (**a**, **b**) The coke bottle shape, bilateral grooves following the linea semilunaris, a median tissue prominence between the costal margin and the pubis, and a new line, corresponding with the existing linea alba vertically divide the mentioned tissue prominence

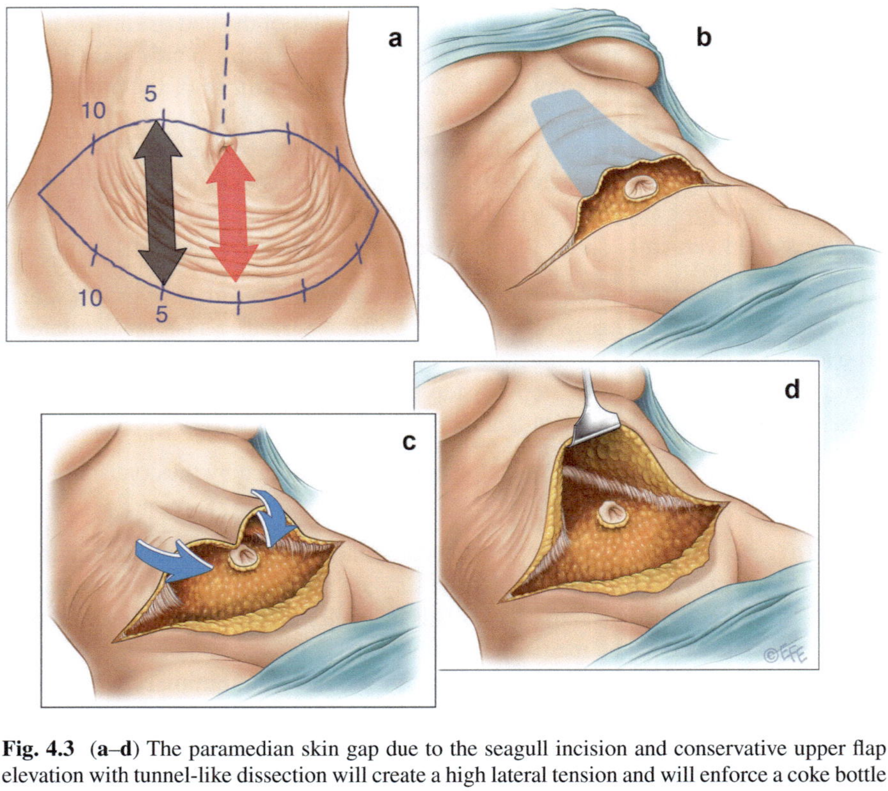

Fig. 4.3 (**a–d**) The paramedian skin gap due to the seagull incision and conservative upper flap elevation with tunnel-like dissection will create a high lateral tension and will enforce a coke bottle shape waist at the time of the closure, while the median convexity of the incision will result in a relative median skin excess from the start of the operation

the lateral abdominal wall. At the time of the closure, both lateral sites of the superior flap will be pulled down and medially to be sutured to lower abdominal wall. Thus, the waist will be pulled medially through these attachments [11].

The paramedian skin gap created by the seagull incision and the lateral skin attachments due to conservative tunnel dissection will together create a high lateral tension and enforce the necessary concavity of the final bottleneck appearance (Fig. 4.3c, d).

2. **The rectus muscle eminence**: The median skin excess is fashioned by:

   A. **Inverse seagull incision**: The median convexity of the seagull incision is designed also to create relative median skin excess from the start of the operation (Fig. 4.3a, *red arrow*).
   B. **The spring sutures**: The authors use multiple triple continuous over-and-over sutures, which resemble a spring, or a helical coil, in order to tighten the fascia in horizontal as well as the vertical plane. Since the expansion of the abdomen due to the musculo-fascial laxity is a threedimensional deformation, which happens in the horizontal as well as the vertical plane, the use of

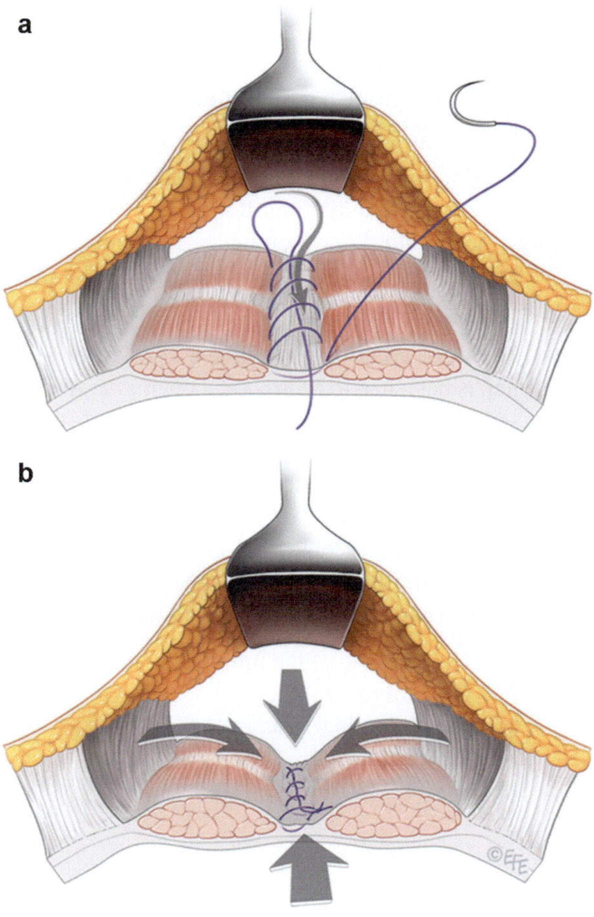

Fig. 4.4 (**a**, **b**) Starting from the upper end of the superior midline tunnel, a triple helix is created with 1-0 polypropylene, as the knot is tied, the fascia is fastened in the horizontal as well as the vertical plane. This will ensure a three-dimensional tightening of the fascia but also shorten the vertical height of the abdominal wall, which in turn will elongate the median part of the superior flap. This excess tissue will be used in order to fashion the false rectus folds

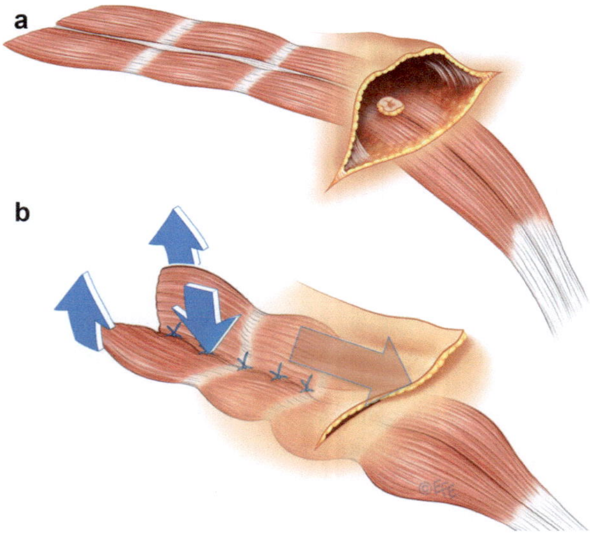

Fig. 4.5 (**a**, **b**) The spring sutures ensure a three-dimensional tightening of the fascia but also shorten the vertical height of the abdominal wall, which in turn will push down and elongate the median part of the superior flap. This excess median tissue will be used in order to fashion the false rectus folds, being divided by the reverse tension of the umbilical anchoring in the later steps

these spring sutures cure the abdominal laxity anatomically (Fig. 4.4a, b). Meanwhile these sutures shorten the vertical height of the abdominal wall elongating the median part of the superior flap. This created relative skin excess and median tissue eminence will be used in order to fashion the rectus folds (Fig. 4.5a, b).

3. **Recreating linea alba**: Once the sufficient amount of median skin excess is created, a central line dividing this excess is fashioned by (a) higher than normal (high positioning) positioning of the umbilicus and (b) anchoring the stalk (umbilical anchoring) and the superior flap to the abdominal fascia with triple sutures.

   A. **High placement of umbilicus**: The new position of the navel on the superior flap is designed to be around 2 cm higher than the projection of the umbilicus stalk on the skin. When this new site is sutured together with the umbilicus to the abdominal wall, the gap between the new umbilicus site and the actual umbilical stalk will be used in order to create a reverse midline tension or an umbilical anchor. The tension of the umbilical anchor will divide the previously created median skin excess into two skin folds, fashioning a double rectus fold illusion (Fig. 4.6a, b).

   B. **Triple sutures**: By triple sutures which incorporate:

      (a) The new site of the umbilicus on the superior flap
      (b) The umbilical stalk
      (c) The abdominal fascia

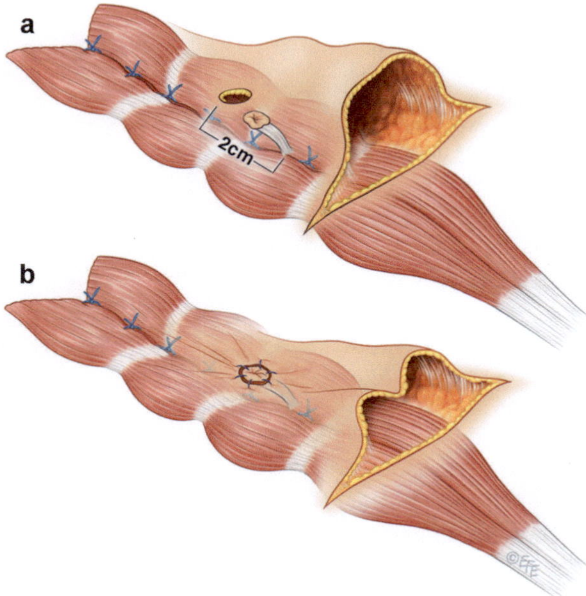

Fig. 4.6 (**a**, **b**) The new site is located around 2 cm higher than the projection of the umbilicus stalk on the skin. This gap between the actual and designed umbilical site will be used in order to create a reverse midline tension or an umbilical anchor. The tension of the umbilical anchor will divide the previously created median skin excess into two skin folds, fashioning the double rectus fold illusion

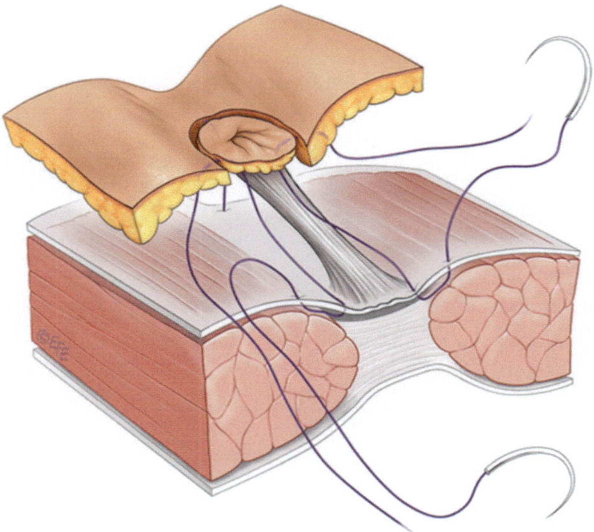

Fig. 4.7 The umbilicus is transposed into the triangular incision and 2-0 Vicryl suture at 3, 6, 9 o'clock positions are placed through the abdominal wall, the base of the umbilical stalk, and the subcutaneous tissue of the superior flap

The midline of the upper flap median skin excess will be pulled down and attached to the fascia without putting any tension on the umbilical stalk (Fig. 4.7).

C. **Umbilical anchoring**: Incorporating the abdominal wall to the umbilical sutures will reduce the tension created on the stalk due to high positioning. This triple

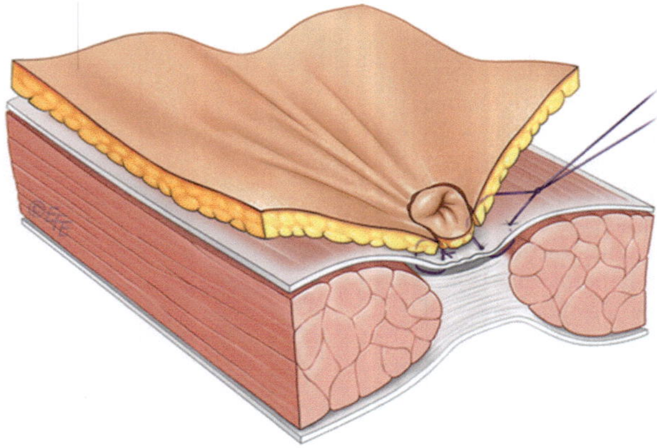

Fig. 4.8 The tension of the umbilical anchor will pull the midline downward, dividing the median skin excess into two skin folds, thus fashioning the double rectus fold illusion

Box: Summary of the Surgical Maneuvers Creating the Anatomical Landmarks

Ideally	Anatomically	Technically	Explanation
Bottleneck	Core muscle concavity with bilateral grooves	(a) Seagull incision (b) Conservative tunnel dissection	Lateral skin gap and median skin excess with high lateral tension
Rectus muscle eminence	Median skin excess	(a) Seagull incision (b) Spring sutures	Median skin excess due to incision and vertical wall shortening
Recreating linea alba	Central reverse tension on the median skin excess	(a) High placement of umbilicus (b) Triple sutures (c) Umbilical anchoring	Repositioning the umbilicus higher and anchoring the skin excess as well as the umbilicus together to the fascia will create the reverse tension dividing the median skin excess in twofolds

suture will pull the epigastric part of the flap thus decreasing tension on the hypogastrium, with much lower risk of suprapubic necrosis. Moreover, this midline reverse tension will divide the previously created median skin excess into two skin folds, fashioning the double rectus fold illusion (Fig. 4.8).

4.5 Conclusion

The ordinary objective of conventional abdominoplasty is to solve the problem of excess abdominal skin but not necessarily to concentrate on a worked-out appearance with the eminences and grooves of the archetypal beautiful tummy. In contrast to this conventional approach, the inverse abdominoplasty with *a midline start, a seagull shape dermolipectomy* with median skin excess and paramedian gap, *horizontal-vertical plication* of the rectus sheath for three-dimensional musculoaponeurotic tightening and adding to the median skin excess, and an *umbilical anchor* with the transposition of the umbilicus to a new more superior location on the abdominal wall skin and recreating line alba would be an extremely effective method to address the problems referred before.

Using these maneuvers, this operation will be a functional surgery with much shorter operation time, but moreover it will be considered a sophisticated beautification procedure.

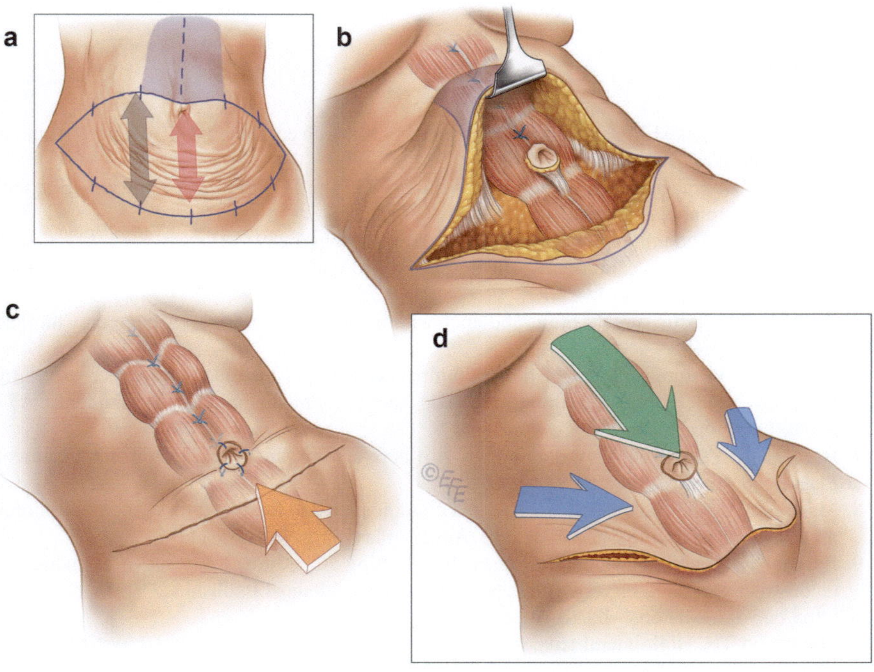

Fig. 4.9 Summary

Points to Remember (Fig. 4.9)

- The coke bottle shape and the bilateral grooves are fashioned primarily by the *seagull incision*, which creates a paramedian skin gap and median skin excess, which is one of the tools to design high lateral tension as well as the final median skin eminence for the rectus illusion. (A)
- Another important surgical maneuver to increase the median vertical skin excess by shortening the vertical abdominal wall is the usage of *spring sutures*. (B)
- The paramedian skin excess in conjunction with the conservative *tunnel dissection* of the superolateral sides of the upper flap help us create the strong high lateral tension necessary for the bottleneck appearance as well as fashion the lateral grooves. (C)
- *High positioning* the belly button is used to create a reverse midline tension. *The triple sutures* between the upper flap, umbilicus and the fascia, the midline of the upper flap median skin excess will be pulled down and attached to the fascia. This tension will divide the previously created median skin excess into two skin folds, thus fashioning a new linea alba and double rectus fold illusion. (D)
- The resulting *umbilical anchor* will improve tightening of the epigastric skin, avoiding residual bulging without putting any tension on the umbilical stalk. It will also decrease the tension on the hypogastrium with much lower risk of suprapubic necrosis

References

1. Baroudi R, Keppke EM, Carvalho CG. Mammary reduction combined with reverse abdominoplasty. Ann Plast Surg. 1979;2(5):368–73.
2. Pacifico MD, Mahendru S, Teixeira RP, Southwick G, Ritz M. Refining trunk contouring with reverse abdominoplasty. Aesthet Surg J. 2010;30(2):225–34.
3. Matarasso A. Abdominolipoplasty. Clin Plast Surg. 1989;16:289–303.
4. Matarasso A. Classification and patient selection in abdominoplasty. Operative Tech Plast Reconstr Surg. 1996;3:7–14.
5. Psillakis JM. Plastic surgery of the abdomen with improvement in the body contour. Clin Plast Surg. 1984;11:465.
6. Pitanguy I. Dermolipectomy of the abdominal wall, thigh, buttocks, and upper extremity. In: Converse J, editor. Constructive plastic surgery. Philadelphia: WB Saunders; 1977. p. 3800–23.
7. Bozola AR, Psillakis JM. Abdominoplasty: a new concept and classification for treatment. Plast Reconstr Surg. 1988;82:983–93.
8. Matarasso A. Abdominoplasty: a system of classification and treatment for combined abdominoplasty and suction-assisted lipectomy. Aesthet Plast Surg. 1991;15:111–21.
9. Baroudi R. Traditional abdominoplasty. In: Grotting JC, editor. Reoperative aesthetic and reconstructive plastic surgery, vol. 2. St Louis: Quality Medical Publishing; 1995.
10. http://en.wikipedia.org/wiki/Abdomen.
11. Lockwood TE. High-lateral-tension abdominoplasty with superficial fascial system suspension. Plast Reconstruct Surg. 1995;96:60.

Chapter 5
The Technique of Inverse Abdominoplasty

Tunc Tiryaki

Box: Summary

- *In inverse abdominoplasty, the procedure starts with a seagull shape midline incision superior to the umbilicus.*
- *First, the flap superior to the umbilicus is elevated and a tunnel is created without lateral dissection to facilitate high lateral tension at the closure.*
- *Then, the umbilicus is separated and the flap inferior to it is dissected towards the mons pubis.*
- *A horizontal-vertical plication of the rectus sheath with helical spring sutures is done for three-dimensional musculo-aponeurotic tightening.*
- *The resulting vertical shortening of the abdominal wall pulls down and elongates the medial part of the skin flap, thus creating significant median skin excess.*
- *During the umbilical transpositioning, the new position of the umbilicus on the abdominal skin is located 2–3 cm superior to the actual stalk position. Fixing the flap as well as the umbilical stalk to the fascia with triple sutures creates an umbilical anchor with a reverse midline pull of the middle part of the superomedial skin flap.*
- *The inferior pull of the anchor divides the median skin excess, thus fashions false rectus muscle folds appearance with a midline valley and lateral tension shadows with a coke bottle shape waist.*
- *Starting with an inferior incision and undermining of the long superior flap is the main reason of the long operative time and difficulty in dissection as well as closure. The inverse start-up facilitates the surgeon to perform the procedure in much shorter time due to shorter flaps superiorly and inferiorly.*
- *Hence the superior start, there is never any need for a T-scar at the closure.*

T. Tiryaki
Department of Plastic Surgery, Cellest Plastic Surgery Center, Istanbul, Turkey
e-mail: drtunctiryaki@gmail.com

K.T. Tiryaki (ed.), *Inverse Abdominoplasty*, DOI 10.1007/978-3-319-39310-0_5

The full abdominoplasty is the most commonly performed method of abdominoplasty because usually abdominal contouring patients present with a combination of significant soft tissue laxity, diastasis recti, abdominal striae and excessive fat accumulation [1].

Inverse abdominoplasty is not a version or type of reverse abdominoplasty. In this technique the surgery starts with a seagull shape supra-umbilical incision and the flaps superior and inferior to the umbilicus are elevated separately. Horizontal-vertical plication and the resulting vertical shortening create significant median skin excess, which is later divided in two folds by high positioning of the umbilicus and resulting reverse tension, thus fashioning false rectus muscle folds appearance with a midline valley and lateral tension shadows with a coke-bottle shape waist. Starting with an inferior incision and undermining of the long superior flap is the main reason of the long operative time and difficulty in dissection as well as closure. The inverse start-up facilitates the surgeon to perform the procedure in much shorter time due to shorter flaps superiorly and inferiorly. Also, there is never a need for a T-scar at the closure [2].

Whatever the technique used, the basic goals of surgery are the removal of the excess loose skin and tightening the underlying musculofascial system employing the least conspicuous incision [3].

5.1 Preoperative Considerations

For a successful outcome, the health status of the patient shall be screened, the medical history taken carefully and any presenting health problem shall be diagnosed and assessed properly before the surgery [4].

Diabetes is an important relative contraindication to abdominoplasty. These patients need careful planning and preoperative monitoring to ensure healthy blood chemistry [5]. Patients with respiratory difficulties may need consultation because the myofascial plication may result in a transient increase in intra-abdominal pressure, which may result in postoperative respiratory difficulties. Smoking is of major concern for all abdominoplasty procedures. Active smokers are at increased risk of ischaemia and skin necrosis, particularly midline in the infraumbilical area above the transverse incision as well as subcutaneous fat necrosis [6].

The abdominoplasty candidates are asked for complete smoking cessation for 3 weeks preoperatively. Still, it is important to note that the associated long-term chronic smoking sequelae can be improved but may not be completely corrected, and these patients continue to be at increased risk for the mentioned problems [7, 8].

Even though a possible pregnancy after abdominoplasty is not a contraindication, patients who consider a future pregnancy are encouraged to have the abdominoplasty be performed following the last pregnancy [9].

Abdominal scars particularly upper abdominal scars, like subcostal cholecystectomy scar from previous operations, should be carefully examined and discussed with the patient of a higher risk of ischaemia and/or necrosis of the skin medially. In these patients, a less aggressive dissection of a mini abdominoplasty with extensive upper plication shall be discussed [4].

Patients who are overweight or who are taking birth control medications or hormone replacement therapy are at increased risk for pulmonary embolism (PE) and deep vein thrombosis (DVT) and this issue should be discussed preoperatively [10, 11].

Such medications should be discontinued for 2 weeks preoperatively in order to reduce the associated risks. In cases where it is not possible to stop these medications, the patient needs to be informed of the increased risk of DVT/PE. A haematology consultation should be considered to evaluate for this.

A family history or any personal incidence of DVT or PE is of even greater concern. Under this circumstance, preoperative laboratory analysis to evaluate the patient's coagulation profile including a factor V Leiden and to search for possible familial tendencies for hypercoagulability is recommended [4].

Skeletal abnormalities such as lumbar lordosis should also be discussed and pointed out to the patient during the consultation since these conditions preclude achieving a flat contour [3].

Box: Preparation for Full Abdominoplasty

- *Smoking cessation/avoidance of nicotine exposure for 2–3 weeks prior to surgery.*
- *Vitamin C for improved wound healing for 2 weeks.*
- *Stop aspirin/other blood thinning products 3 weeks before surgery.*
- *Abstain from all dietary/herbal supplements and herbal teas for 2 weeks.*
- *Special clotting tests if there is a personal or family history.*
- *Cardiology and respiratory clearance if needed.*
- *Shower with a gentle antimicrobial soap in the morning of surgery.*

Box: Relative Contraindications for Abdominoplasty

- *Continuing smoking*
- *Diabetes mellitus*
- *Serious vasculitis*
- *Wound healing disorders*
- *Immunodeficiency*
- *Necessity of continuous usage of blood coagulation inhibitors*
- *Significant history of pulmonary or deep vein thrombosis*
- *Serious medical problems*

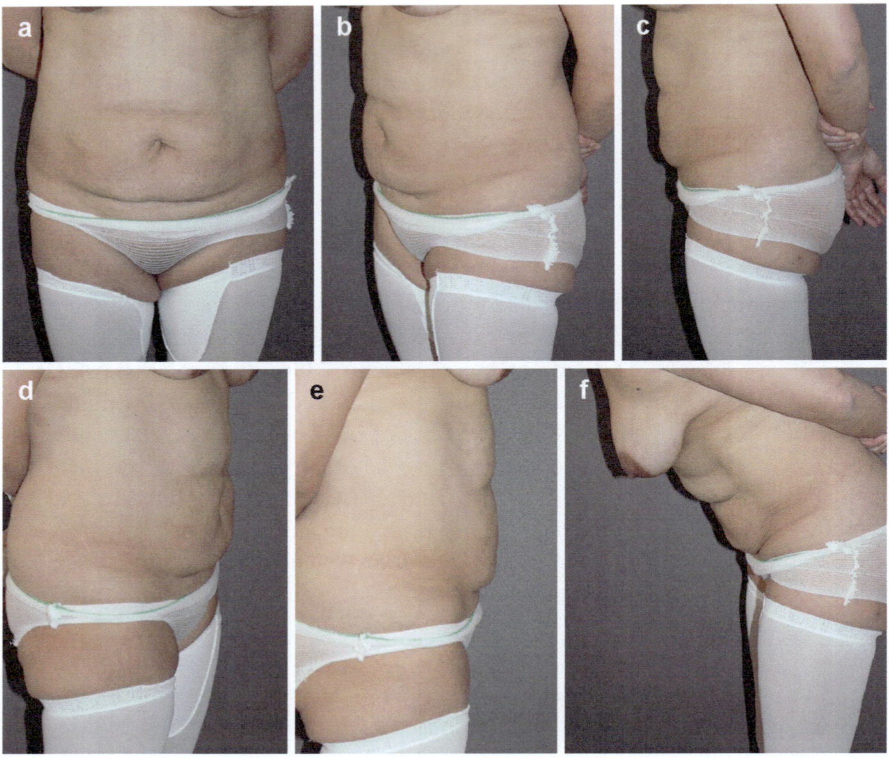

Fig. 5.1 (**a–f**) Preoperative pictures are taken usually in six cardinal views. If a complementary liposuction is going to be performed, a posterior view is added. All pictures include the area from infra-mammary folds to mid-thigh, demonstrating the abdominal contour, waistline, the extent of the abdominal wall laxity and skin to be resected

5.2 Surgical Technique

5.2.1 Preoperative Photography and Markings

Initially, preoperative photographs are taken in anterior, bent, right and left oblique and right and left lateral views. Patients are marked in a standing position to delineate the areas for liposuction and skin incisions, wearing their preferred undergarments to confine the final incision within the boundaries of her clothing (Fig. 5.1).

The marking starts with a midline drawing from the xiphoid to umbilicus and to the anterior vulvar commissure with the patient standing, which will serve also as a reference line to facilitate symmetry and to better appreciate any excess of tissue on either side. Two paramedian vertical lines are also drawn 5–6 cm off the midline symmetrically (Fig. 5.2).

Holding the pannus upwards, a curvilinear incision is marked in the natural inferior skin fold, extending in length slightly beyond the lateral skin folds with the patient

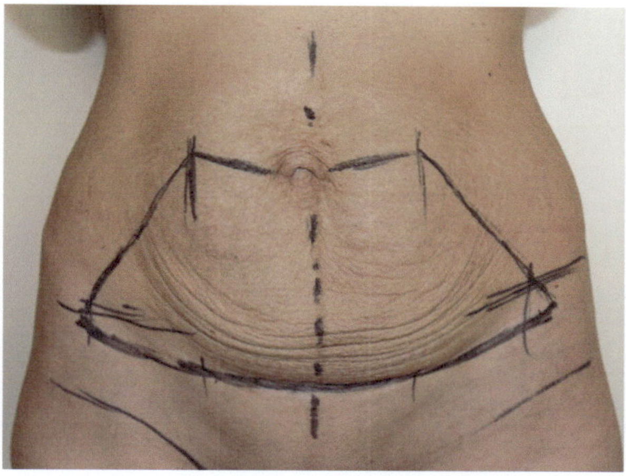

Fig. 5.2 The marking starts with a midline drawing from the xiphoid to the umbilicus and to the anterior vulvar commissure with the patient standing. Two paramedian vertical lines are also drawn 5–6 cm off the midline symmetrically. Holding the pannus upwards, a curvilinear incision is marked in the natural inferior skin fold. A seagull shape superior line is designed at the level of the upper border of the belly button. This superior horizontal line is first drawn gently upwards, peaking up around 5–6 cm away on both sides from the midline at the paramedian lines, then curves downwards towards the lateral endings of the inferior incision line, usually close to the anterior superior iliac spines

in a lateral hip-flexed position. A seagull shape superior line is designed at the level of the upper border of the belly button through the both lateral sides. This superior horizontal line is drawn gently upwards, peaking up around 5–6 cm away on both sides from the midline at the paramedian lines, then curves downwards towards the lateral endings of the inferior incision line, usually close to the anterior superior iliac spines.

The amount of the skin to be removed is double-checked by the surgeon grasping the skin and confirming that the upper and lower incisions meet. The definitive markings for the real amount of tissue resection are done on the operative table. The patients are dressed with thromboembolic deterrent stockings before they are called to the operating room (OR).

Points to Remember

- Six different cardinal views are necessary in preoperative photography.
- The incision shouldn't extend beyond the bikini lines.
- The skin excess above the umbilicus should be observed *(or checked)* preoperatively.
- A seagull shape incision is planned in order to create the necessary paramedian skin gap and the following inferomedial tension.

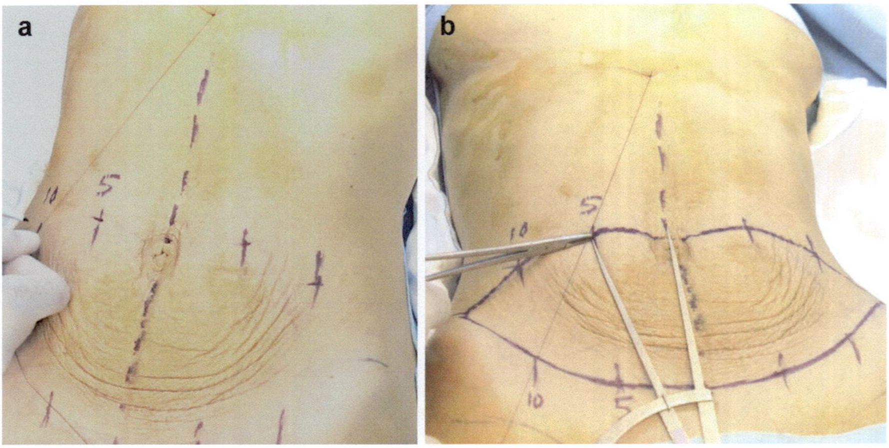

Fig. 5.3 (**a**, **b**) The seagull incision: Note that the bilateral curves of the upper marking will result in a relative paramedian skin gap. At the operation table with the patient in the supine position, the previous markings are reverified using a 2-0 silk suture placed in the midline at the level of the xiphoid and vertical parallel lines at 5, 10 and 15 cm. The symmetry of the upper seagull shape incision and the lower incision are ascertained

5.2.2 Positioning and Planning

The surgery is usually performed under general anaesthesia. If multiple operations are performed like facial procedures or breast interventions, the authors usually perform the abdominal surgery as first procedure except of liposuction.

In the OR, the operating table is checked to insure that it can be flexed prior to induction of anaesthesia. The patient is placed in a supine position with silicone pillows under the knees to prevent nerve compressions during the surgery.

Afterwards, the symmetry of the body and the arms is verified, a rolled towel of 5–10 cm diameter is positioned behind the back of the patient at the level of the scapulae in order to decrease the unnatural backwards leaning of the thorax on the operating table and the arms are loosely secured by wrapping them with gauze. A Foley catheter is inserted, sequential pneumatic compression devices are placed and if indicated anticoagulants are used.

To ensure symmetry a 2-0 silk suture is placed in the midline at the level of the xiphoid. Vertical parallel lines at 5, 10 and 15 cm are drawn and a symmetrical upper incision line with a seagull shape is obtained at the crossing of the vertical lines using the silk suture. The same drawing is performed for the lower planned incision (Fig. 5.3a, b).

Preoperative preparations end by infiltrating 0.5 ml of 1:1000 epinephrine and 10 ml of 2 % lidocaine solution in 100 ml saline solution directly through the incision lines.

Points to Remember

- The operating table is checked to insure that it can be flexed prior to induction of anaesthesia.
- A rolled towel is placed under the back at the level of each scapula bones to mimic natural standing position.
- Vertical parallel lines at 5, 10 and 15 cm are drawn and a symmetrical upper incision line with a seagull shape is obtained at the crossing of the vertical lines using the silk suture. The same drawing is performed for the lower planned incision.

5.2.3 Inverse Incision and Superior Flap Elevation

First, the upper incision above the umbilicus is made. A slightly bevelled incision through the cutis is made through the superior seagull shape marking, while pulling the skin only downwards in order to achieve proper cutting angle (Fig. 5.4).

Then, the blade bevels more to lie at 30° to the surface of the flap, so the Scarpa's fascia portion of the flap is about 1 cm shorter than the skin portion. This manoeuvre will ensure the scar-edge elevation and an optimal skin closure with good scar healing at the end of the surgery. The bilateral upwards curves of the incision are designed to create a relative paramedian skin gap and median skin excess.

The supra- and subscarpal fat is transversed until the surgeon reaches the abdominal wall. The large vessels are suture-ligated and the rest of the dissection is done by electrocautery or harmonic scalpel, leaving the fine areolar tissue and their lymphatics over the fascia. This is thought to diminish the rate of seroma formation [12].

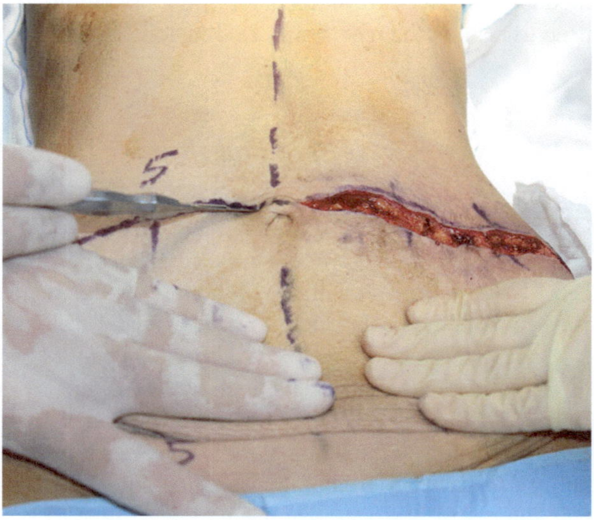

Fig. 5.4 The slightly bevelled incision while pulling the skin only downwards will ensure the scar-edge elevation and an appropriate skin closure with good scar healing at the end of the surgery

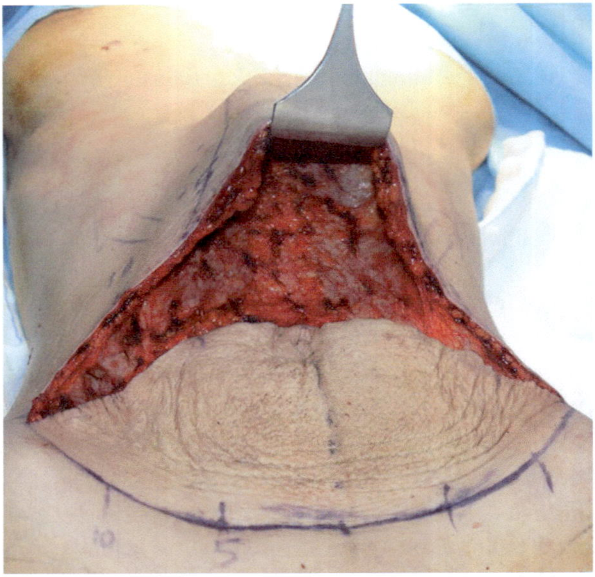

Fig. 5.5 The lack of lateral dissection and the previously created paramedian skin gap will ensure an extra pull towards the midline and create a defined coke bottle appearance at the end of the procedure

The upper abdominal flap is undermined up to the xiphoid, resembling a narrow midline tunnel, maintaining the intercostal blood supply sufficiently to achieve rectus muscle repair and anterior sheath plication (Fig. 5.5).

The lack of the lateral dissection and the minimal dissection of costal margins creates a lateral tension at the closure of the skin. This, in conjunction with the tension created by the paramedian skin gap due to the seagull incision will pull the waist towards the midline and help the surgeon create a coke bottle appearance [13].

The median convexity of the seagull incision helps also to create a relative median skin excess from the start of the operation. This tissue excess will later be used to fashion the rectus muscles illusion.

5.2.4 Navel Dissection and Inferior Flap Elevation

Once the upper flap is elevated, a cold towel is placed into the dissected tunnel and around the flap in order to decrease capillary bleeding (Fig. 5.6). An upside-down heart-shape is drawn around the umbilicus with a diameter of 1–1.5 cm, and then it is freed from the lower skin flap with 15 blade scalpel (Fig. 5.7a–c).

Once the navel is separated, the surgeon changes his position from the right side of the patient to the left side, which will make the lower dissection much easier for right-handed surgeons (Fig. 5.8). The lower flap dissection is performed in the same way downwards to the inguinal region. Extra attention is paid to the haemostasis for perforators around the umbilicus, which are numerous and one of the most important sources of postoperative haematoma (Fig. 5.9). The inferior dissection is continued past the planned level of the final closure in order to lift the thigh region and to rejuvenate the inguinal area as well (Fig. 5.10).

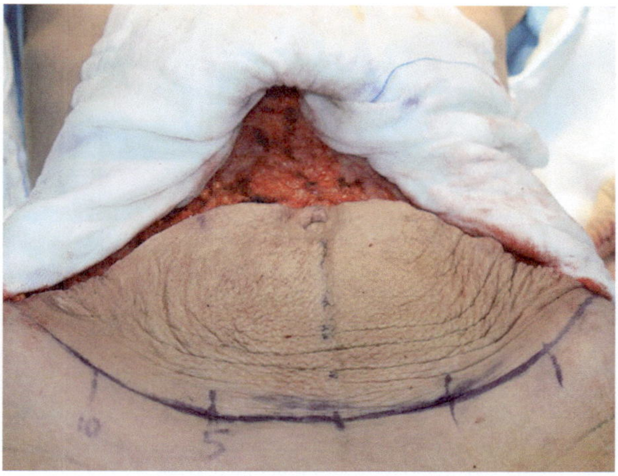

Fig. 5.6 Cooling of the superior flap in order to reduce the blood loss

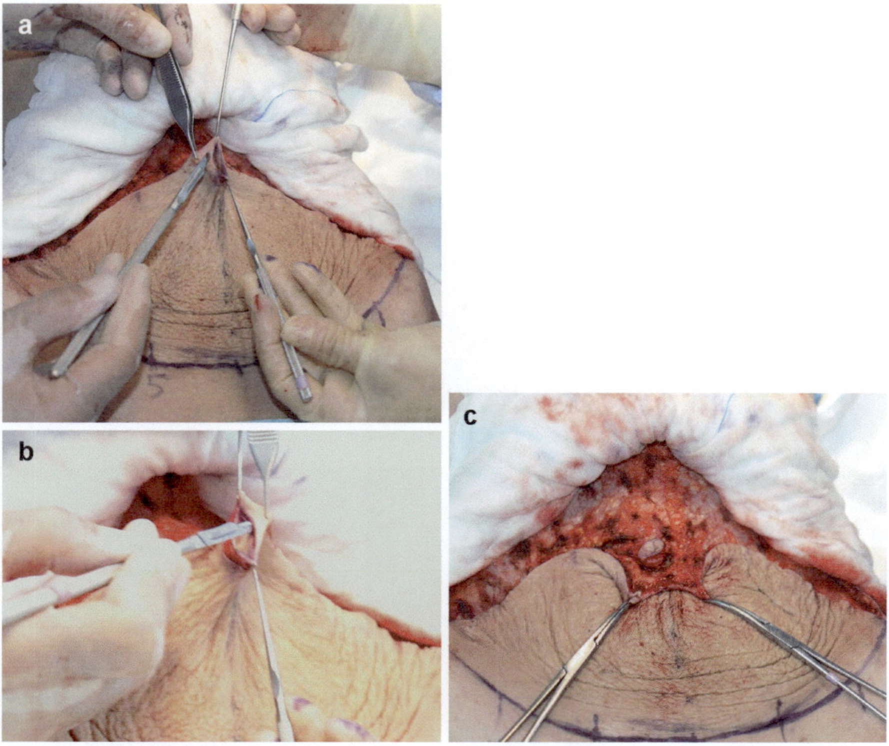

Fig. 5.7 (**a**–**c**) A heart shape is drawn with a diameter of 1–1.5 cm and the umbilicus is freed from the lower flap

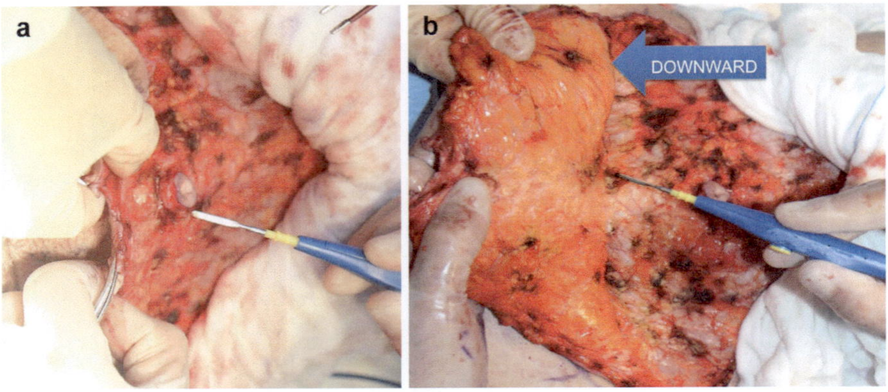

Fig. 5.8 (**a**, **b**) The surgeon changes his position from the right side of the patient to the left side, which will make the lower dissection much easier for right-handed surgeons. (The opposite is valid for left-handed surgeons, who shall start from the left and change to right for lower dissection.)

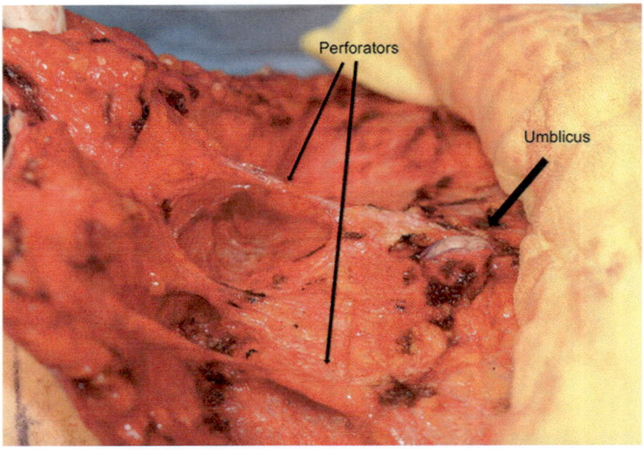

Fig. 5.9 Extra attention is paid to the haemostasis for perforators around the umbilicus, which are numerous and one of the most important sources of postoperative haematoma

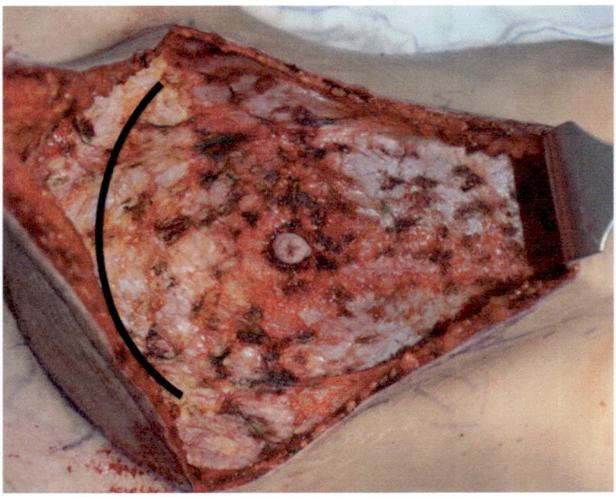

Fig. 5.10 Lower flap dissection finished. Note that dissection is continued past the planned level of the final closure, in order to lift the thigh region

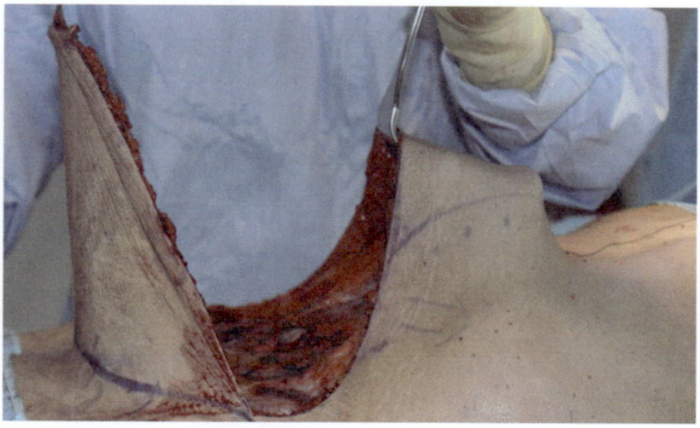

Fig. 5.11 Upper and lower flaps elevated in much shorter time and minimal effort due to the ease of dissecting two shorter superior and inferior flaps instead of one long superior flap

In this fashion, the dissection of both flaps is completed very fast and easy because of short flap length superiorly and inferiorly as well as the excellent control over the surgical area. It is also comfortable for the assistant to retract the flaps and to control the haemostasis (Fig. 5.11).

Points to Remember

- Bevelled incisions for reduced closure tension and better scar healing.
- Inverse seagull incision without lateral dissection for creating the lateral skin gap.
- Upper flap elevation without lateral dissection to increase the lateral tension.
- Navel dissection and lower flap elevation past the planned closure line.
- A very fast and easy dissection because of short flap length and excellent control.

5.2.5 *Spring Sutures: Horizontal-Vertical Plication*

It is important to note that the expansion of the abdomen due to the "musculofascial" laxity is a three-dimensional deformation, which happens in the horizontal as well as the vertical plane. A definitive treatment of this condition necessitates a horizontal-vertical plication of the abdominal wall. The authors use a triple continuous over-and-over suture, which resembles a spring, or a helical coil, in order to tighten the fascia in horizontal as well as the vertical plane. The horizontal-vertical plication serves two purposes. First of all it is curing the three dimensional abdominal laxity in an anatomical way. Second, it shortens the abdominal wall vertically and elongates the median part of the superior flap.

To do this, the diastasis is noted and an ellipse is marked on the anterior rectus sheath from the xiphoid to the pubis. The widest portion of the ellipse is located at the level of the navel, with a width of around 6–10 cm according to the laxity (Fig. 5.12).

Starting from the upper end of the superior midline tunnel, a triple helix is created with 1-0 polypropylene. These buried sutures start with taking a bite at the left lateral edge of

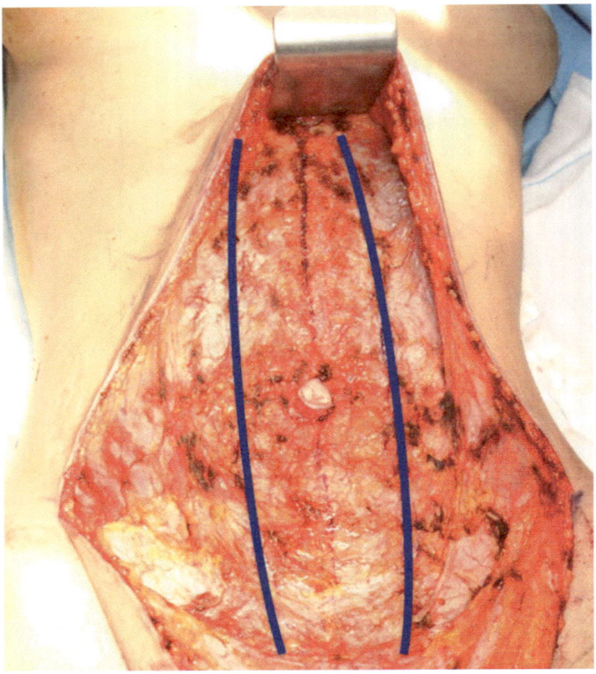

Fig. 5.12 The diastasis is noted and an ellipse is marked on the anterior rectus sheath from the xiphoid to the pubis, the widest portion being around 6–10 cm according to the laxity

the diastasis, then the right side, repeating three times to create a triple helical loop around the tread itself, fashioning a spring of Prolene (Fig. 5.13a–e). As the knot is tied, the fascia is fastened in the horizontal as well as the vertical plane (Fig. 5.14a, b). These separate triple helical spring sutures are used as many as needed above and then below the umbilicus down to the pubis all along the midline. This will ensure a three-dimensional tightening of the fascia but also shorten the vertical height of the abdominal wall, which in turn will elongate the median part of the superior flap. This will increase the tissue excess which was initially created by the median convexity of the seagul incision. This tissue eminence will later be used to fashion the rectus muscle folds illusion (Fig. 5.15a, b).

Points to Remember

- The expansion of the abdomen is a three-dimensional deformation, which shall be dealt with a three-dimensional treatment.
- A definitive treatment of this condition necessitates a horizontal-vertical plication of the abdominal wall.
- The authors use *spring sutures*, triple continuous over-and-over sutures, which resemble a spring or a helical coil.
- The uses of horizontal-vertical spring sutures are twofold: repairing abdominal laxity anatomically and elongating the median part of the superior flap which will be used to create false rectus folds illusion
- Another advantage of the vertical muscle sheet plication is that it allows the surgeon to excise more skin

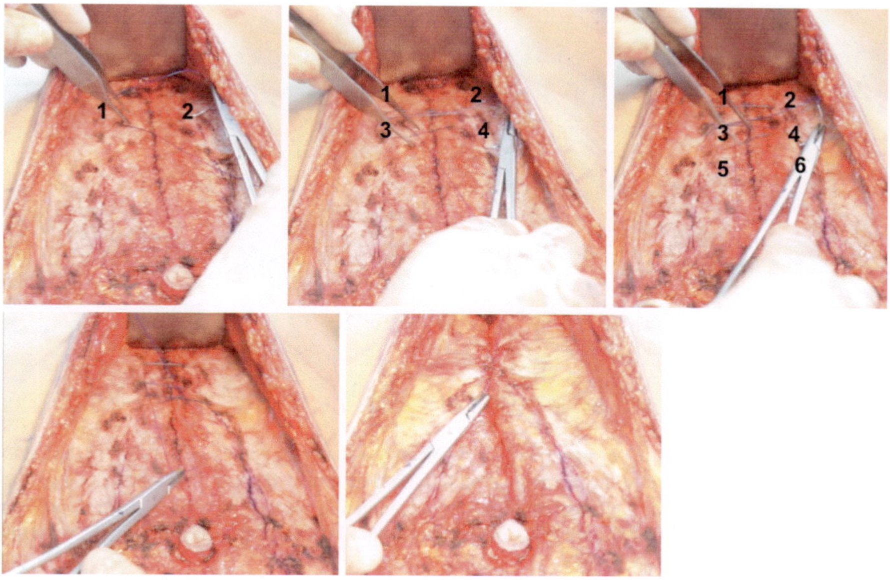

Fig. 5.13 (**a–e**) Starting from the upper end of the superior midline tunnel, triple helix sutures are created with 1-0 polypropylene for the plication of the abdominal wall. These buried sutures start with taking a bite at the left lateral edge of the diastasis, then the right side, repeating three times to create a triple helical loop around the tread itself, fashioning a spring of Prolene. When tying the knot, the abdominal wall will be plicated not only in the horizontal but also in the vertical plane

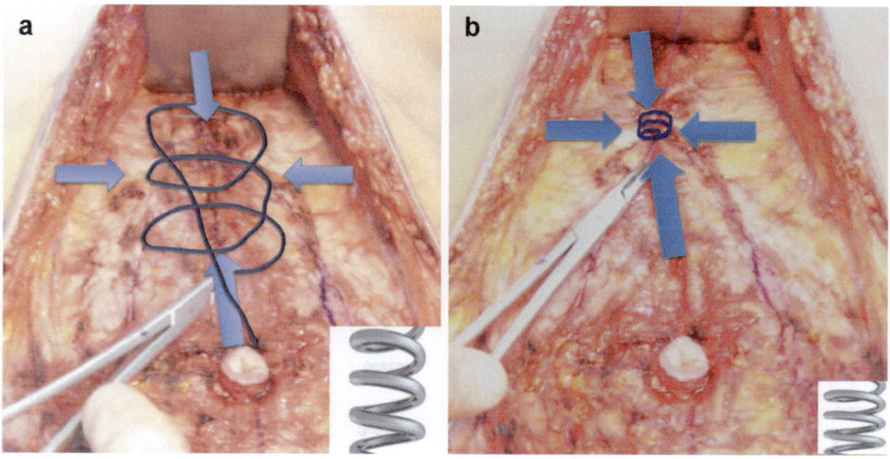

Fig. 5.14 (**a**, **b**) Starting from the upper end of the superior midline tunnel, a triple helix is created with 1-0 polypropylene, as the knot is tied, the fascia is fastened in the horizontal as well as the vertical plane. The vectors show the directions of the abdominal wall tightening

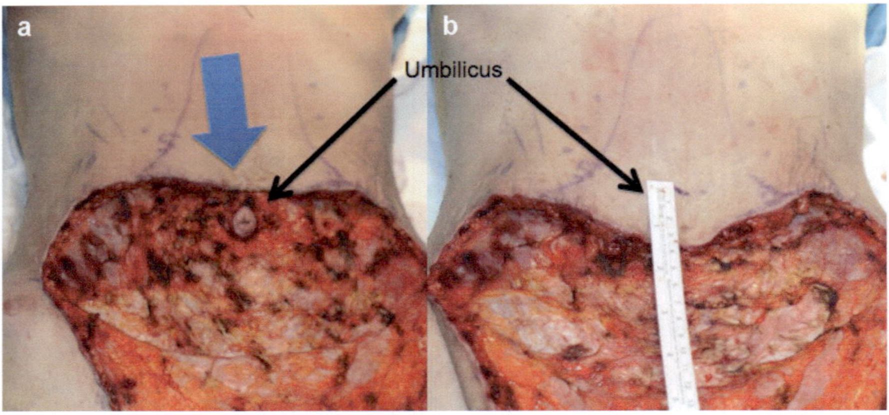

Fig. 5.15 (**a**, **b**) The triple sutures ensure a three-dimensional tightening of the fascia, but also shorten the vertical height of the abdominal wall, which in turn will push down and elongate the median part of the superior flap (Vector). This excess median tissue will be used in order to fashion the false rectus folds, being divided by the reverse tension of the umbilical anchoring in the later steps

5.3 Subfascial Anaesthesia

Meticulous haemostasis is ensured after the plication. About 40 cc of 0.25 % bupivacaine solution is prepared and around 10 cc of this solution is injected per quadrant just beneath the external fascia of the rectus and the external oblique muscles, with blunt needles to anaesthetise the regional nerves to the abdominal muscles. The trajectory of the needle should be visualised by translucency through the fascia to ensure the proper depth of the injection [14]. This local anaesthetic injection immensely decreases the patient's need for narcotics for the whole postoperative period (Fig. 5.16).

Points to Remember

- 10 cc of 0.25 % bupivacaine solution is injected *per quadrant* immediately beneath the external fascia.
- This immensely decreases the patient's postoperative pain and need for narcotics for the *whole* postoperative period.

5.3.1 Inferior Midline Triangle

After the infiltration is done, the table is flexed to 30–40°, and the upper flap is pulled downwards below the lower flap to ensure that the superior flap length is sufficient for the planned pannus excision (Fig. 5.17a, b). The inferior marking is realigned and 10 cm of the mid-portion cutaneous incision is performed; however, the incision is not continued all through the subcutaneous tissue. A 5–5 cm triangle

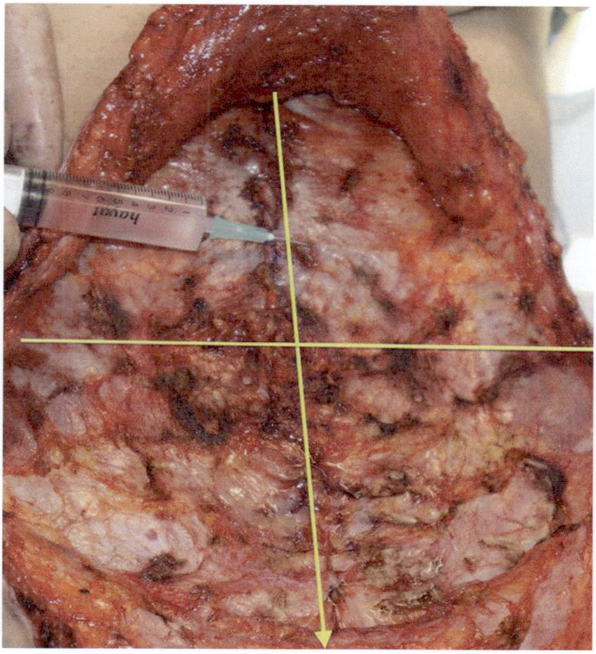

Fig. 5.16 Ten cc of local aesthetic solution is injected per quadrant just beneath the external fascia of the rectus and the external oblique muscles with blunt needles to anaesthetise the regional nerves to the abdominal muscles. The trajectory of the needle should be visualised by translucency through the fascia to ensure the proper depth of the injection

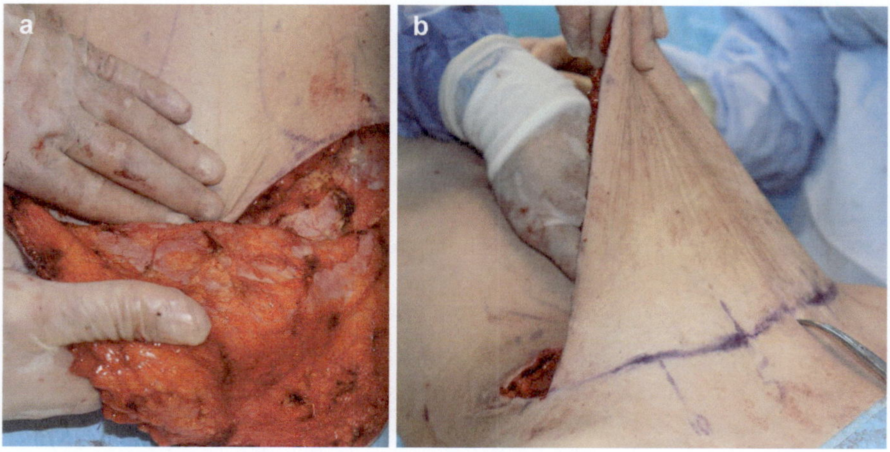

Fig. 5.17 (**a**, **b**) The tab. is flexed to 30–40°, and the upper flap is pulled downwards below the lower flap to ensure that the superior flap length is sufficient

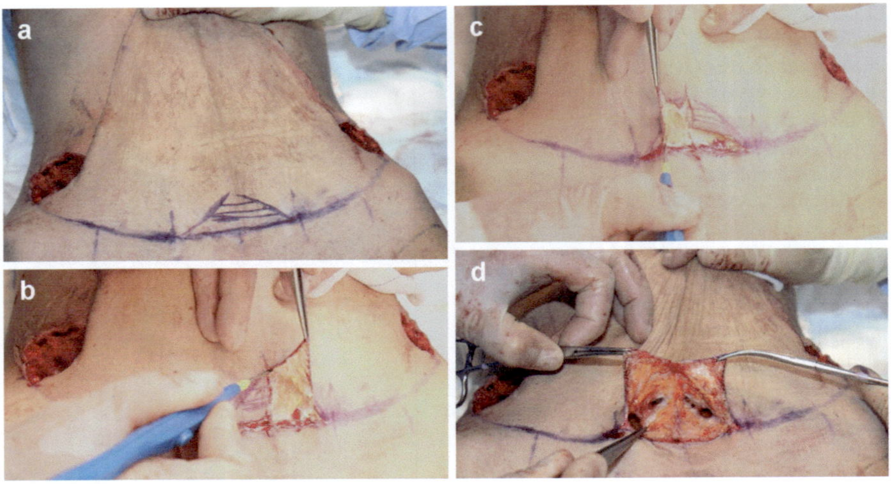

Fig. 5.18 (**a–d**) The inferior marking is checked and a midline 10 cm cutaneous incision is performed through the dermis. However, the incision is continued through the subcutaneous tissue. A 5–5 cm triangle of subcutaneous fat tissue is deepithelialised and left attached as a fat flap to the pubic skin then the rest of the inferior flap is divided in two lateral flaps. The middle triangular subcutaneous flap will be used to fill the natural umbilical stalk defect at the closure

of subcutaneous fat tissue is deepithelialised and left attached as a fat flap to the median pubis skin, while the inferior flap is divided in two lateral flaps. The middle triangular subcutaneous flap will be used to fill the natural umbilical stalk defect at the upper flap edge (Fig. 5.18a–d).

5.3.2 New Umbilical Site

One of the key manoeuvres for this operation is positioning the new umbilical site. In order to locate the new navel position, the lower edge of the superior flap is sutured temporarily to the pubis.

Two rules are used to determine the site of the new umbilicus:

(a) The site must be located around 2 cm higher (high positioning) than the projection of the umbilicus stalk on the skin. This gap between the new umbilicus and the umbilical stalk will be used in order to create a superior tension (Fig. 5.19a, b). After fixing the stalk and the skin flap to the abdominal wall, this gap between the new umbilicus site and the umbilical stalk will create a reverse midline tension or an umbilical anchorage.
(b) The site must be located around 10 cm above the pubic incision.

The new higher umbilical site is marked accordingly and a skin triangle with edges of 1.5 cm is excised (Fig. 5.20). At the back of the flap, a circular *defatting* of the subcutaneous tissue around the new navel area is performed in order to mimic the natural slope around the navel.

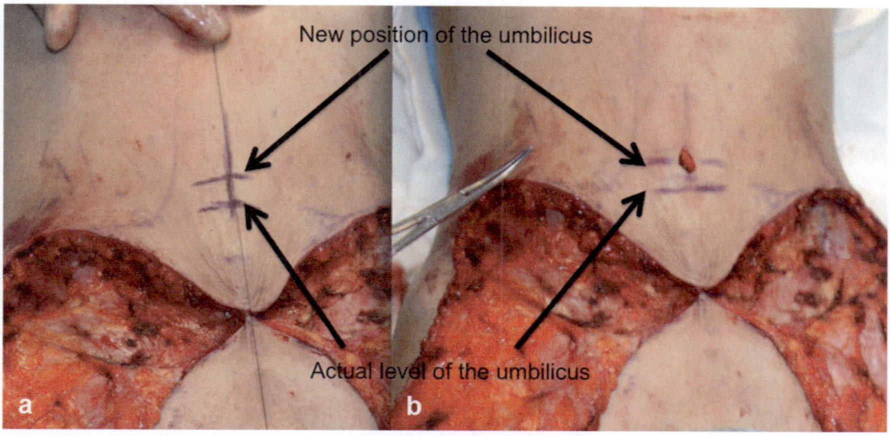

Fig. 5.19 (**a**, **b**) The new site is located around 2 cm higher than the projection of the umbilicus stalk on the skin. This gap between the new umbilicus and the umbilical stalk will be used in order to create a reverse midline tension, or an umbilical anchorage

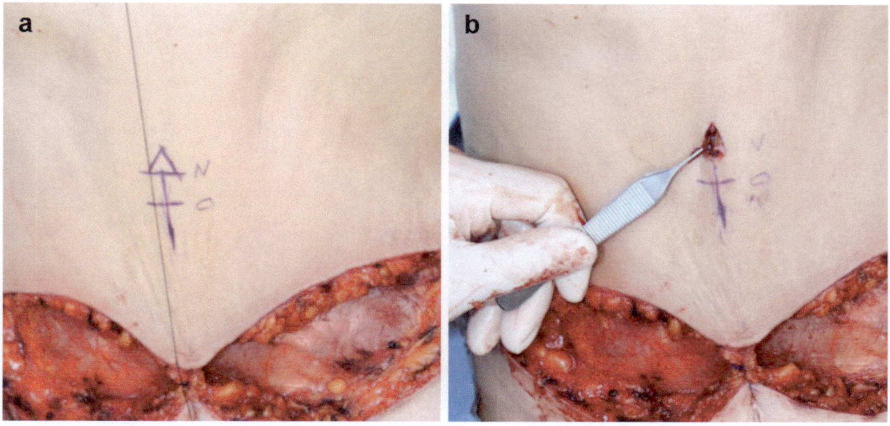

Fig. 5.20 (**a**, **b**) Location and shape of the umbilical triangle

5.3.3 Umbilical Anchorage with Triple Sutures

The umbilicus is transposed into the triangular incision, and 2-0 Vicryl sutures at 3, 6 and 9 o'clock positions are placed first through the abdominal wall, then the base of the umbilical stalk and finally the subcutaneous tissue of the superior flap, suturing the umbilicus as well as the superior flap to the periumbilical abdominal wall (Fig. 5.21).

Incorporating the abdominal wall and the stalk to the abdominal wall anchor sutures reduces the tension created on the stalk due to high positioning. This triple suture also pulls the epigastric part of the flap thus decreasing tension on the hypogastrium, with much lower risk of suprapubic necrosis [15].

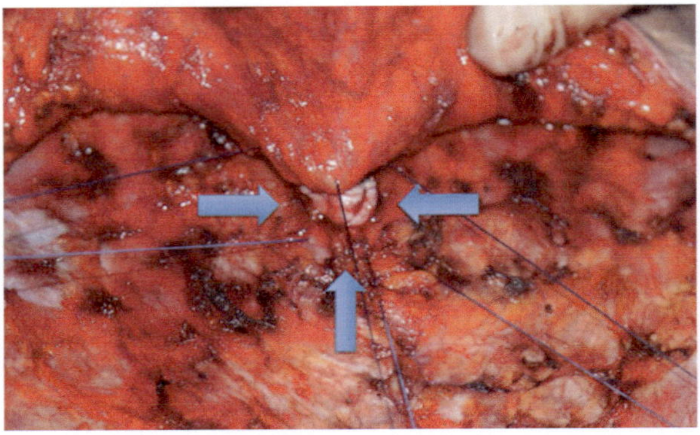

Fig. 5.21 The umbilicus is transposed into the triangular incision, and 2-0 Vicryl suture at 3, 6, 9 o'clock positions (Vectors) are placed through the abdominal wall, the base of the umbilical stalk and the subcutaneous tissue of the superior flap

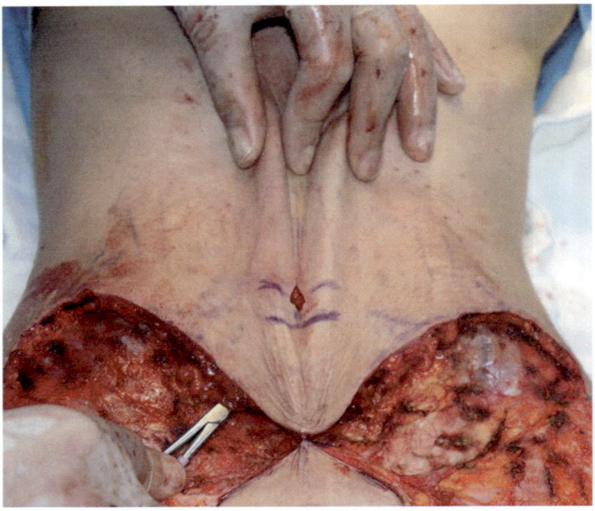

Fig. 5.22 The tension of the umbilical anchorage will divide the previously created median skin excess into two skin folds, fashioning the double rectus fold illusion

But most importantly, the reverse midline tension due to the gap between the newly designed umbilicus site and the umbilical stalk will divide the previously created median skin excess into two skin folds, fashioning the double rectus fold illusion (Fig. 5.22).

Points to Remember

- The umbilical anchorage will improve tightening of the epigastric skin, avoiding residual bulging.
- Decreased tension on the hypogastrium, with much lower risk of suprapubic necrosis.
- The excess skin is transferred to the hypogastrium.
- Incorporating the abdominal wall to the umbilical sutures reduces the tension created on the stalk due to high positioning.
- These sutures will anchor the umbilicus as well as the superior flap to the abdominal wall in order to create a reverse midline tension, dividing the previously created median skin excess into two skin folds, thus fashioning the double rectus fold illusion.

5.3.4 Excision and Scar Shortening

Resection of the abdominoplasty flap is done after the umbilicus is secured to its new location. A temporary suture is placed at the midline between the edge of the superior flap and the lower flap (Fig. 5.23a). To remove the redundant skin, the superior skin edges on both sides of the suture are pulled down below the inferior flaps and the preoperative markings are verified. If there is a necessity, the marking are realigned according to the skin excess and the inferior skin flaps are resected with careful haemostasis of the edges. This bilateral pull will help to elevate the thigh, adding a rejuvenation of this area (Fig. 5.23b, c). The lateral apices of the wound, the region where dog-ears typically occur, may require suction assisted or direct lipectomy to provide a smooth contour.

After the excision is done, a final inspection for haemostasis is performed prior to closure. Special attention is paid for the inferior epigastric artery and vein. Once the haemostasis is ensured, the realignment of the superior and inferior flaps are planned.

First, using a 2-0 Vicryl suture, the previously prepared triangular subcutaneous flap is sutured to the abdominal wall in order to fill the umbilicus defect of the superior flap. This dramatically reduces the typical midline hollowness at suture site. Then, the superior flap is sutured to this subcutaneous tissue flap.

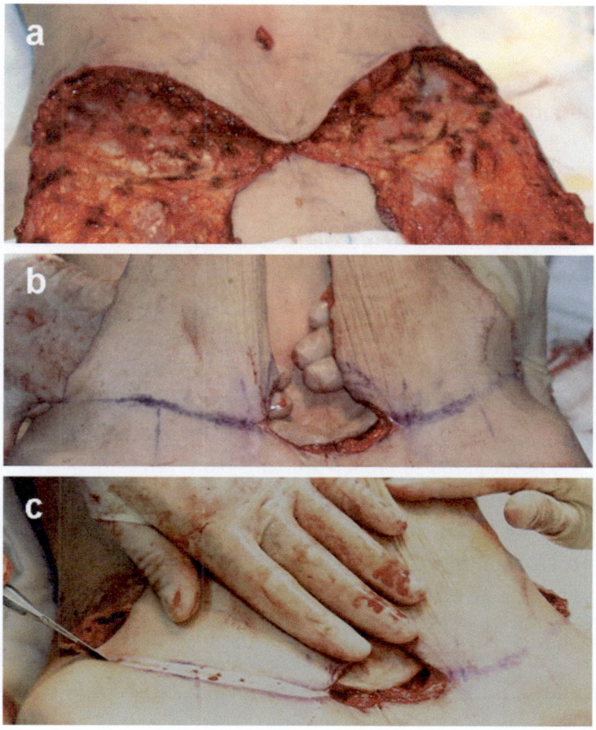

Fig. 5.23 (**a–c**) Resection of the abdominoplasty flap is done after the umbilicus is secured to its new location. A temporary suture is placed at the midline and to remove the redundant skin, the superior flap edges are pulled down bilaterally below the inferior flaps and the preoperative markings are verified. If there is a necessity, the marking are realigned according to the skin excess and the inferior skin flaps are resected with careful haemostasis of edges

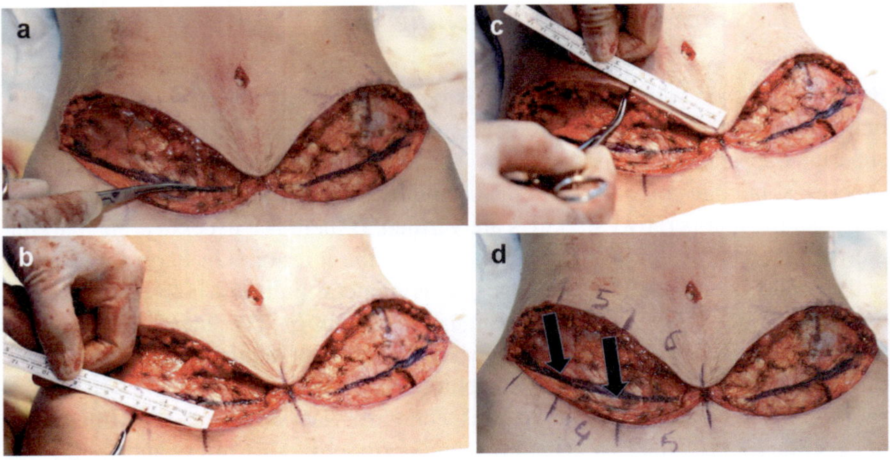

Fig. 5.24 (**a**) In order to prevent the incision line to drift upwards, a symmetrical marking is done on the abdominal wall where both flaps are going to be secured. (**b–d**) Since the upper flap has a tendency to drift laterally and also the incision line is longer than the inferior flap edge, there is a need to pull the superior flap medially and shorten the incision length. This is obtained by marking the vertical closure lines differently on both flaps. At the upper flap edge, 6th, 5th, 4th centimetres and, on the lower edge, 5th, 4th, 3rd centimetres are marked symmetrically from midline. Suturing these vertical marks together, the upper incision is shortened symmetrically fitting the lower and the upper flap ends are pulled medially. This creates a bilateral medial advancement, which helps to enhance the final shape of the waist

Once the midline is secured, a symmetrical horizontal marking is done on the abdominal wall where both flaps are going to be secured to prevent the incision line to drift upwards (Fig. 5.24a).

Since the upper flap has a tendency to drift laterally and also the superior incision line is longer than the inferior flap edge, there is a need to pull the superior flap medially and shorten the incision length. This is obtained by marking the vertical closure lines differently on both flaps. At the upper flap edge, 6th, 5th, 4th centimetres and, on the lower edge, 5th, 4th, 3rd centimetres are marked symmetrically from midline (Fig. 5.24b–d). Suturing these vertical marks together using 2-0 Vicryl, the upper incision is shortened symmetrically fitting the lower, and the upper flap ends are pulled medially. This creates a precise bilateral medial advancement, which helps to enhance the final shape and contour of the waist.

The incision is closed starting from lateral towards medial, and any redundancy is compensated towards the midline decreasing any dog-ear formation. Once the Scarpa's fascia is approximated and fixed to the abdominal wall at the level of the previous marking, the symmetry of the scar is ensured and any superior drift is prevented. These sutures also take the tension off of the skin closure and allow for fine skin closure (Fig. 5.25a).

For the superficial closure, two 3-0 bidirectional barbed sutures are used in the superficial fat layer and the dermis on either side of the midline in a running fash-

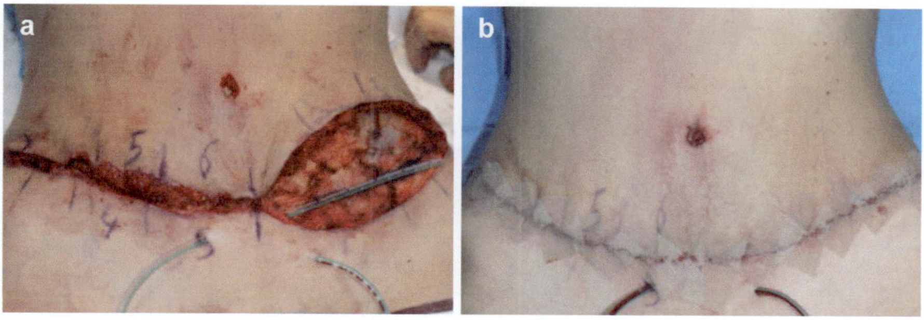

Fig. 5.25 (**a**, **b**) The incision is closed by 2-0 Vicryl sutures, starting from lateral towards medial, and any redundancy is compensated towards the midline decreasing any dog-ear formation. This medial advancement of the upper abdominal flaps provides a significant improvement in the final shape of the waist. Scarpa's fascia is approximated and fixed to the abdominal wall at the level of the previous marking, thus ensuring the symmetry of the scar as well as preventing the superior drifting using 2-0 Vicryl sutures. These sutures also take the tension off of the skin closure and allow for fine skin closure

ion [14]. The umbilicus is closed with running intradermal 4-0 Monocryl. The umbilicus is packed with Xeroform gauze and the incision line is steri-stripped (Fig. 5.25b).

Two multi-perforated drains are placed beneath the abdominal flap in a criss-cross fashion to avoid kinking, exiting in the pubic skin without any fixation. Finally, before the anaesthesia is ended, horizontal splinting tape dressings are placed around the abdomen followed by an elastic girdle (Fig. 5.26a–d).

Points to Remember

- Resection of the abdominoplasty flap is done after the umbilicus is secured to its new location and flaps are sutures together in the midline to ensure proper skin excess calculation.
- The pull of the lower flap will help to elevate the thigh, adding a rejuvenation of this area.
- In order to keep the incision line low at the desired height, a symmetrical marking is done on the abdominal wall where both flaps are going to be secured.
- Since the upper flap has a tendency to drift laterally and also the incision line is longer than the inferior flap edge, there is a need to pull the superior flap medially and shorten the incision length.
- The incision is closed starting from lateral towards medial, and any redundancy is compensated towards the midline decreasing any dog-ear formation.
- Scarpa's fascia is approximated and fixed to the abdominal wall at the level of the fascia marking, ensuring symmetry and prevention of superior drift.
- Two multi-perforated drains are placed beneath the abdominal flap in a criss-cross fashion.

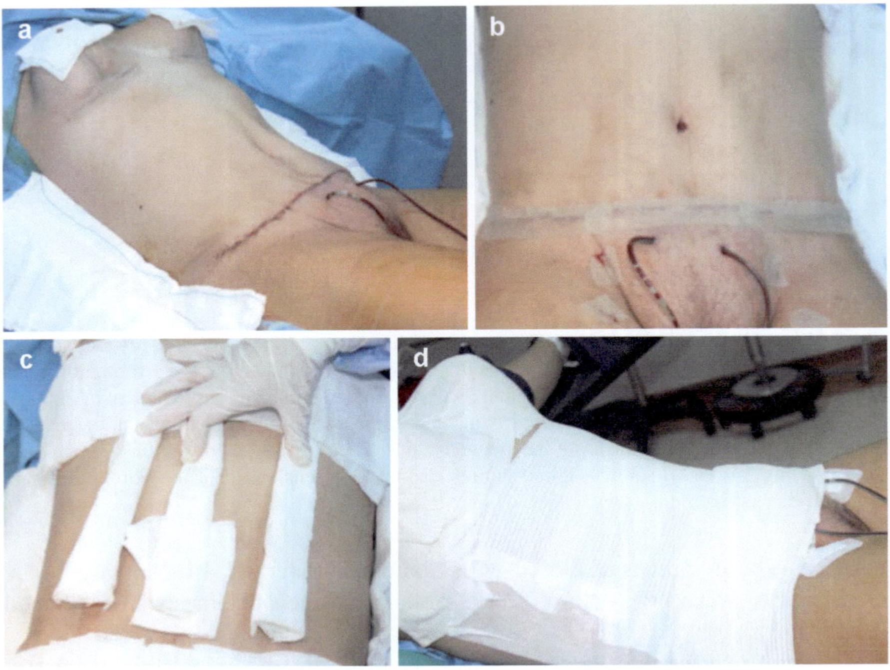

Fig. 5.26 (**a–d**) Two multi-perforated drains are placed beneath the abdominal flap in a criss-cross fashion to avoid kinking, exiting in the pubic skin without any fixation. The umbilicus is packed with Xeroform gauze, the incision line is steri-stripped, vertical lines of the created folds are reinforced by roll gauze, after hypoallergic banding, horizontal splinting tape dressings are placed around the abdomen followed by an elastic girdle

5.4 Postoperative Care

At the end of the procedure, the patients are warmed with warming blankets. An elastic compression binder is applied and worn continuously for at least 3 weeks except of showering. The patients are given intravenous fluids and antibiotics and clear liquid diet for the first postoperative day. Supportive stockings and pneumatic boots are kept on until the patient is walking [12].

The patient is encouraged to be in a semi-sitting position the night of the surgery with immediate and progressive ambulation in a semi-flexed position. The drains are removed when the drainage declines to less than 30 cc per 24 h and after the drains are removed the patient is sent home usually on the first day of the surgery.

The patients are discharged with oral antibiotics/anti-inflammatory medication and are instructed to stay slightly flexed and to refrain from vigorous activity. They are encouraged to walk regularly and move the lower extremities while in bed to help reduce the chance of DVT/PE. Drinking plenty of liquid is advised and the abdominal binder is worn at all times in the first 48 h [4].

The first follow-up visit is after 48 h, where all the splinting tapes are removed, and the patient is encouraged to take full shower. The patients usually go back to

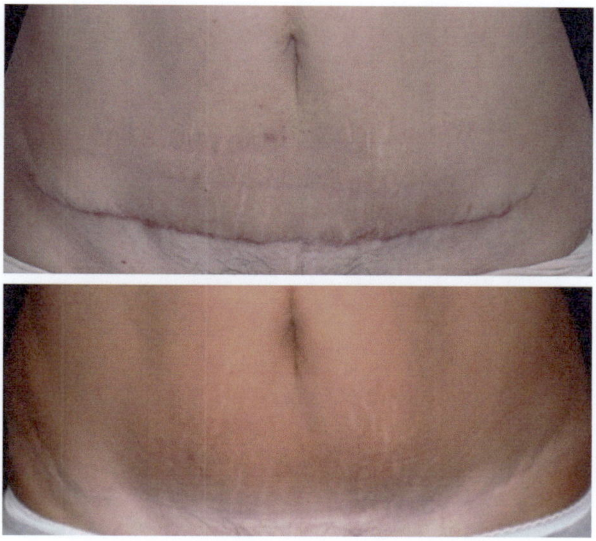

Fig. 5.27 The scar after 2 months and after 2 years

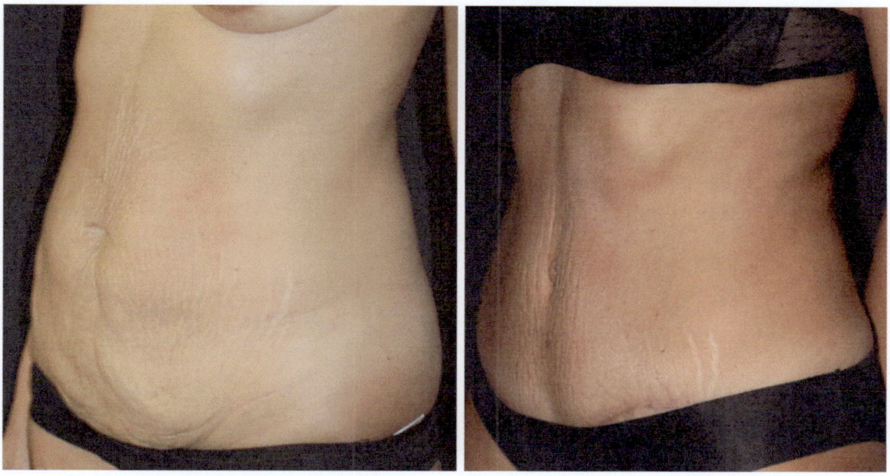

Fig. 5.28 Supraumbilical striae will persist after abdominoplasty

work after the first week. Full daily activity is resumed in 2–3 weeks after surgery and cardio training without abdominal workout is allowed after 4 weeks.

Two weeks after the surgery, the patients are advised to start using silicon bands over the scars. The scar colour and width significantly improves after the first postoperative year (Fig. 5.27). One important note is to inform the patients, who have severe striae over the umbilicus, that these supraumbilical striae even though pulled lower will continue to exist (Figs. 5.28, 5.29, 5.30, 5.31, 5.32, 5.33, 5.34 and 5.35).

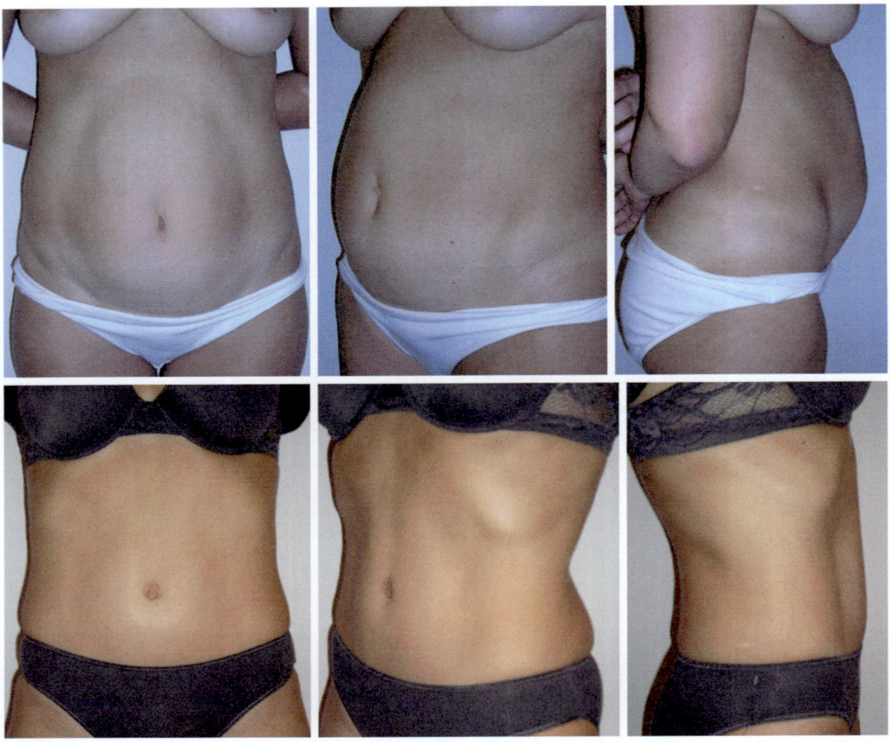

Fig. 5.29 A 42-year-old woman after two children. The patient has relatively good skin quality and body habits. Preoperatively, there was no excess adiposity but significant abdominal wall laxity. She underwent full inverse abdominoplasty with horizontal-vertical myofascial plication without any liposuction. The postoperative two years photographs show the powerful reduction of the waist only with abdominoplasty and false rectus folds

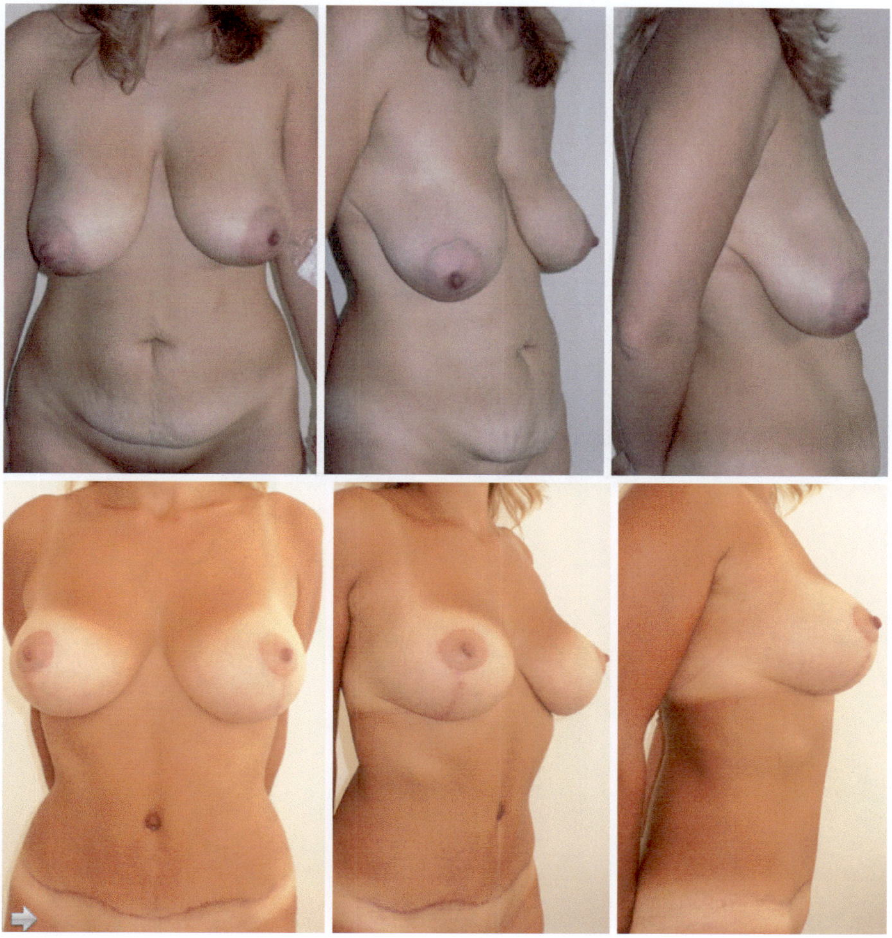

Fig. 5.30 A 50-year-old woman, mother of three children. She underwent a full inverse abdominoplasty with horizontal-vertical myofascial plication and reduction mastopexy. Postoperatively, the patient demonstrates significantly improved contour of the abdomen, false rectus folds, thinning of the trunk with coke bottle shape

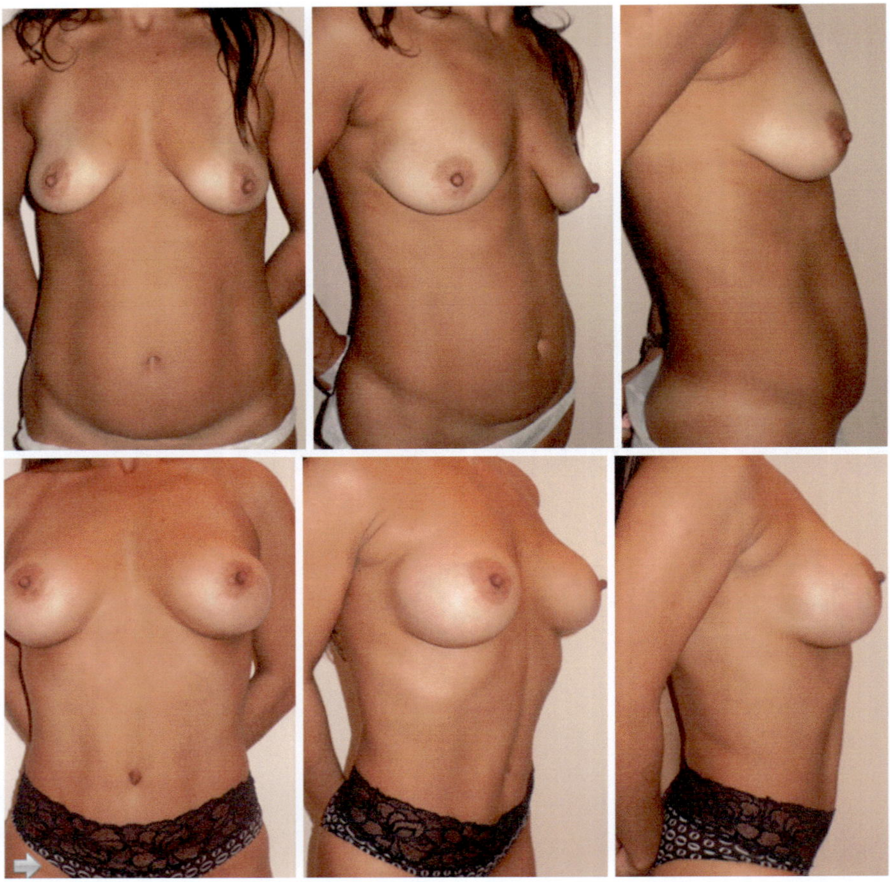

Fig. 5.31 A 43-year-old woman, mother of two children. She underwent a full inverse abdominoplasty with horizontal-vertical myofascial plication and augmentation mammoplasty. Postoperatively, the patient demonstrates the typical coke bottle shape with false rectus folds

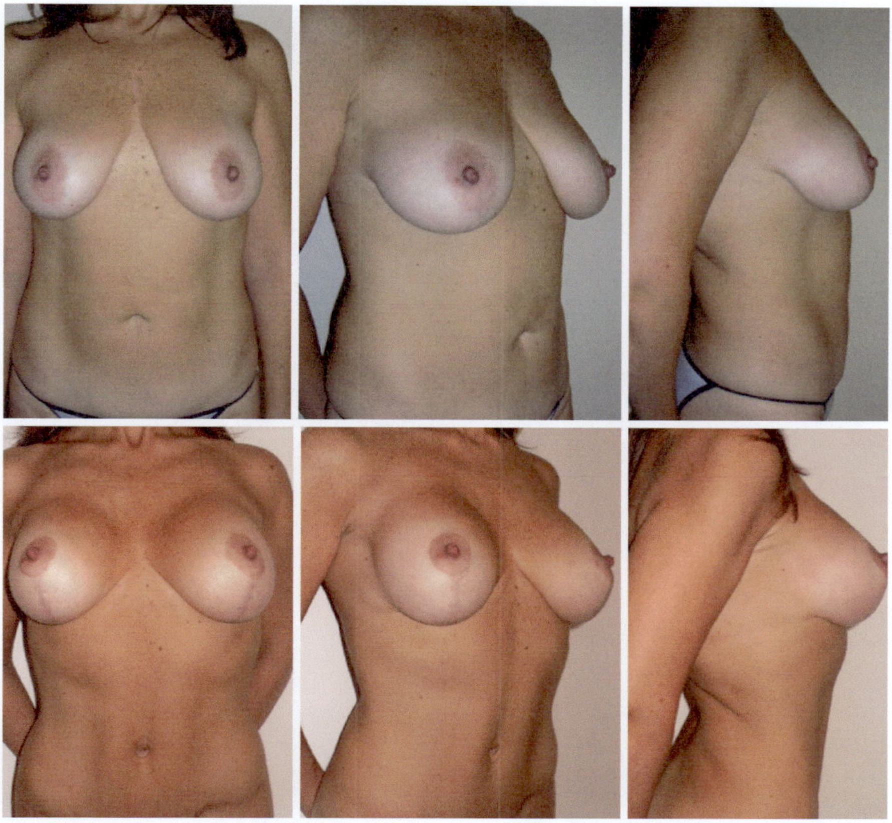

Fig. 5.32 A 45-year-old woman. This patient demonstrated poor waistline definition and contour secondary to abdominal wall laxity with moderate adiposity. There was moderate soft tissue laxity and her skin quality was fair. After inverse full abdominoplasty with horizontal-vertical myofascial plication without any concurrent liposuction, the patient demonstrates dramatically improved abdominal contour, waistline and silhouette with false rectus folds

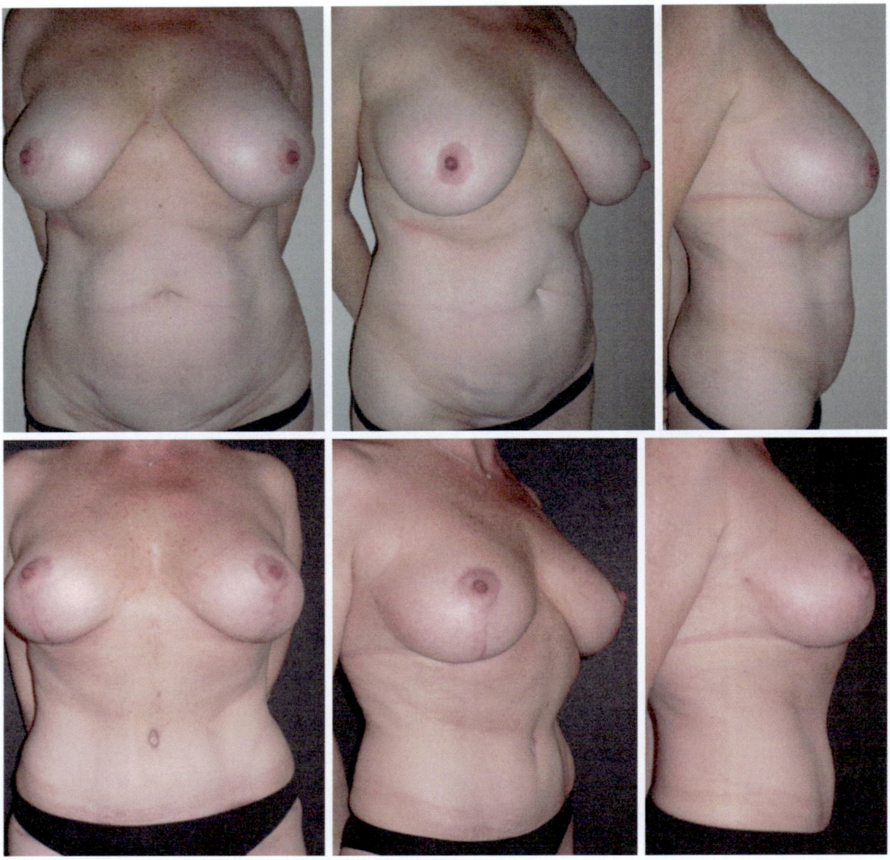

Fig. 5.33 A 55-year-old woman. This patient demonstrated poor waistline definition and contour secondary to abdominal wall laxity with moderate to significant adiposity. After reduction mastopexy and inverse full abdominoplasty with horizontal-vertical myofascial plication without any concurrent liposuction, the patient demonstrates dramatically improved abdominal contour, waistline and silhouette with false rectus folds

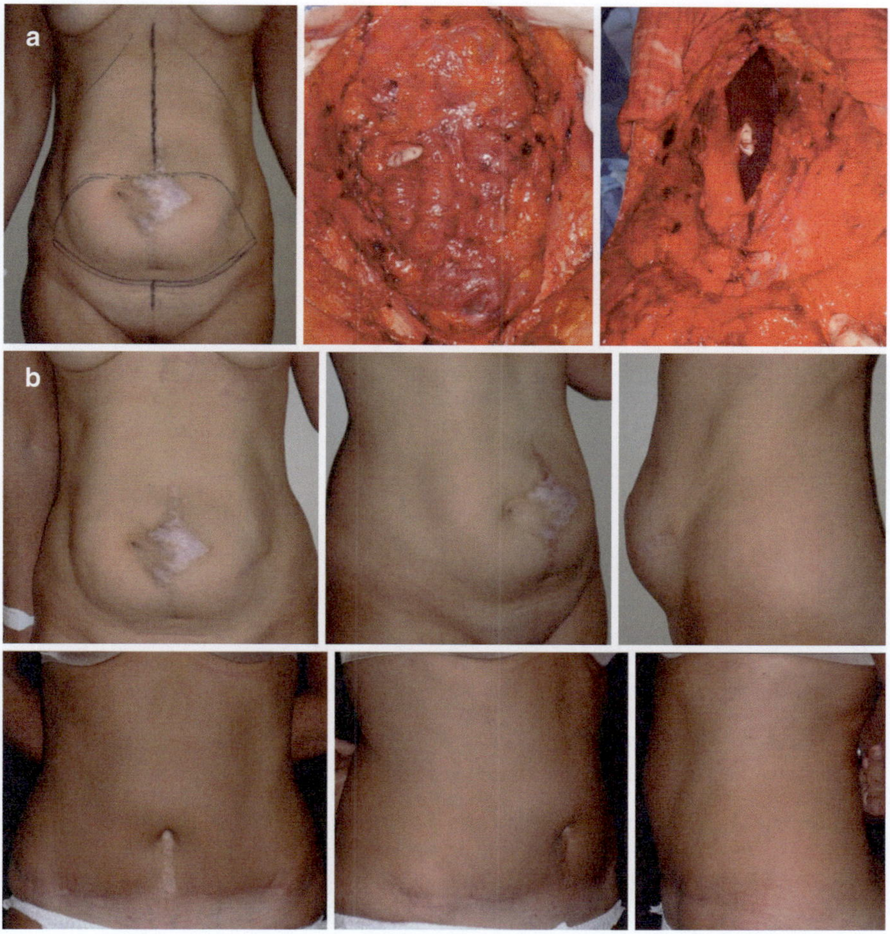

Fig. 5.34 (**a**) A 47-year-old woman after having three abdominal surgeries with life-threatening complications. Abdominal wall integrity was totally lost with the umbilicus pulled towards right. Intestinal movements were palpable and visible in the midline with the peritoneum immediately below the scar area. The inverse start made the planning of the closure and the dissection dramatically easier. A 20 cm horizontal gap was observed after the dissection. The intra-abdominal organs were dissected from the scar tissue, the umbilicus was centralised and the abdominal defect was repaired with polypropylene mesh. (**b**) The postoperative photographs show a full recovery of the eventration

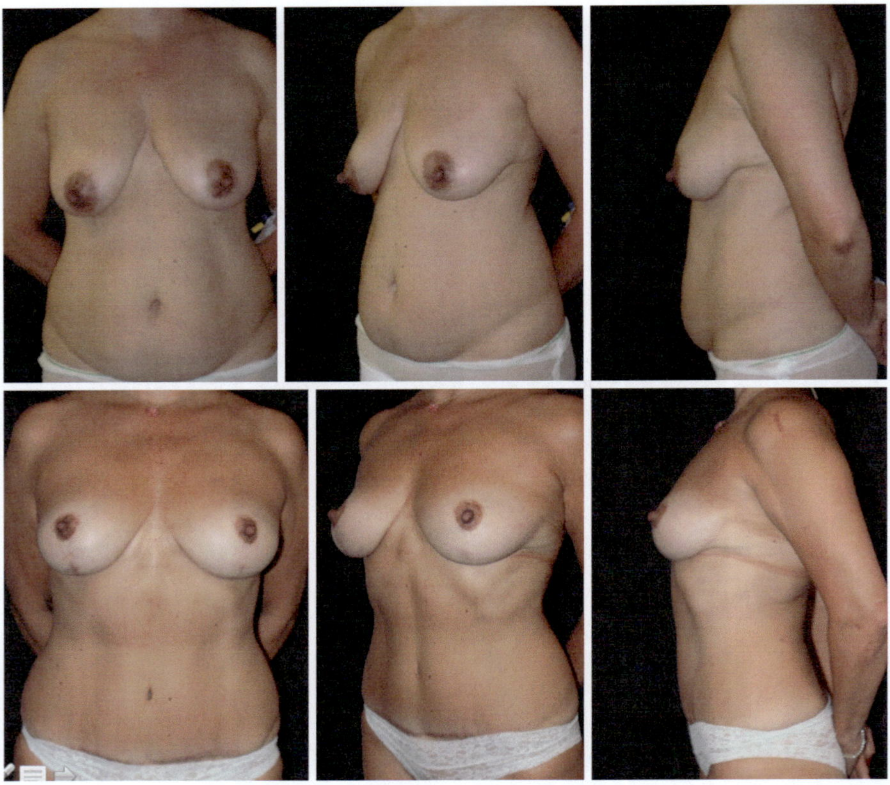

Fig. 5.35 A 53-year-old woman. Moderate skin tonus, wall laxity and significant adiposity. After mastopexy augmentation, inverse full abdominoplasty without liposuction, the patient demonstrates significant improvement of the abdominal contour, waistline and silhouette with false rectus folds

Box: Postoperative Instructions for Full Abdominoplasty

- Use the incentive spirometer frequently.
- Avoid smoking or exposure to nicotine-containing products.
- Drink plenty of fluids: 2 l/day is the goal.
- Move legs frequently while resting and walk regularly.
- Continue to take medications as instructed.
- Maintain a partially flexed position at the waist for the first 1 week.
- Wear the abdominal binder for 3 weeks at all times except for showering.
- Shower on the second day after the first visit.
- Steri-strips are taken away on the first week of visit.
- No driving for 1 week.
- Easy walking after 2 weeks.
- No vigorous activity for 3 weeks.
- No abdominal training for 3 months.

References

1. Matarasso A, Swift RW, Rankin M. Abdominoplasty and abdominal contour surgery: a national plastic surgery survey. Plast Reconstruct Surg. 2006;117:1797.
2. Matarasso A. Abdominolipoplasty. Clin Plast Surg. 1989;16:289–303.
3. Steven GW, Matarasso A. Abdominolipoplasty: classification and patient selection. In: Shiffman MA, Mirrafati S, editors. Aesthetic surgery of the abdominal wall. Berlin/New York: Springer; 2005. p. 70–86, 289–303.
4. Hunstad JP, Repta R. Atlas of abdominoplasty, vol. 7. Philadelphia: Elsevier; 2009. p. 55–75.
5. Guyuron B, Raszewski R. Undetected diabetes and the plastic surgeon. Plast Reconstruct Surg. 1990;86:471.
6. Manassa EH, Hertl CH, Olbrisch RR. Wound healing problems in smokers and nonsmokers after 132 abdominoplasties. Plast Reconstruct Surg. 2003;111:2082.
7. Hensel JM, Lehman Jr JA, Tantri MP, et al. An outcomes analysis and satisfaction survey of 199 consecutive abdominoplasties. Ann Plast Surg. 2001;46:357.
8. Krueger JK, Rohrich RJ. Clearing the smoke: the scientific rationale for tobacco abstention with plastic surgery. Plast Reconstruct Surg. 2001;108:1063.
9. Borman H. Pregnancy in the early period after abdominoplasty. Plast Reconstruct Surg. 2002;109:396.
10. Blickstein D, Blickstein I. Oral contraception and thrombophilia. Curr Opin Obstet Gynecol. 2007;19:370.
11. van Vlijmen EF, Brouwer JL, Veeger NJ, et al. Oral contraceptives and the absolute risk of venous thromboembolism in women with single or multiple thrombophilic defects: results from a retrospective family cohort study. Arch Intern Med. 2007;167:282.
12. Ramirez O, Robertson KM, Khan A. Abdominoplasty technique: a personal approach. In: Shiffman MA, Mirrafati S, editors. Aesthetic surgery of the abdominal wall, vol. 10. Berlin/New York: Springer; 2005. p. 115–20.
13. Lockwood TE. High-lateral-tension abdominoplasty with superficial fascial system suspension. Plast Reconstruct Surg. 1995;96:60.
14. Matarasso A. Traditional abdominoplasty. Clin Plast Surg. 2010;37:415–437.
15. Louarn CL, Pascal JF. The High-Superior-Tension Technique: Evolution of Lipoabdominoplasty. Aesth Plast Surg. 2010; 34:773–81

Chapter 6
Inverse Mini-abdominoplasty

Tunc Tiryaki and Asu Deniz Burhanoglu

6.1 Introduction

Abdominoplasty candidates can visit plastic surgeons with a wide variety of problems. While some have serious skin excess and abdominal wall laxity after heavy weight loss, many have less drastic complaints of weight and skin quality related to changes from aging, pregnancy, and childbirth. Therefore, each patient needs to be carefully assessed, and based on the characteristics of each individual, the proper type of contouring procedure shall be chosen [1]. The assessment must evaluate the component irregularities of the abdominal wall, which consist of varying degrees of adiposity, loose or redundant skin, and laxity of the musculofascial units [2].

When:

(a) The mentioned problems affect majorly the supra-umbilical area.
(b) The whole of the abdomen is affected.
(c) The skin length superior from the umbilicus to the xyphoid is shorter than the distance from the umbilicus to the pubis.

A full abdominoplasty is indicated. However, this procedure almost always necessitates general anesthesia and is associated usually with a higher degree of discomfort and convalescence, frequently requiring an overnight stay in the hospital [3].

On the other hand, the patients who present with limited deformities confined to the central lower abdomen can be treated effectively with a mini-abdominoplasty and a full-length abdominal wall plication. This procedure usually encompasses a shortened scar and a smaller skin excision and is ideal for younger patients with lower abdominal soft-tissue laxity that is not significant enough to allow us to perform a full

T. Tiryaki (✉)
Department of Plastic Surgery, Cellest Plastic Surgery Center, Istanbul, Turkey
e-mail: drtunctiryaki@gmail.com

A.D. Burhanoglu
Mare Clinic, Istanbul, Turkey

K.T. Tiryaki (ed.), *Inverse Abdominoplasty*, DOI 10.1007/978-3-319-39310-0_6

Table 6.1 A simple classification system for decision-making process

Class	Visceral fat	Skin elasticity	Musculofascial tonus	Treatment
Class I	−+	Good	Good	Liposuction
Class II	−+	Good	Moderate	Endoscopic abdominoplasty
Class III	−+	Average	Moderate	Mini-abdominoplasty
Class IV	−+	Poor	*	Inverse abdominoplasty
Class V	++	*	*	No surgery

*Insignificant

abdominoplasty skin resection. Depending on the original location of the navel, with smaller skin resections, the umbilical position can be left unchanged [2, 4].

6.2 Patient Selection

As shown on the chart and Table 6.1, the crucial parameter in decision-making process is the skin quality, meaning the amount and the location of skin excess and the existence of stretch marks [5, 6].

If the mentioned skin problems affect majorly the infraumbilical area, a reverse mini-abdominoplasty and a full-length abdominal wall plication with or without floating umbilicus might be enough to get an excellent result. Similarly, if the skin quality is generally good but the existing wall laxity is considerable, again, a mini-abdominoplasty together with or without liposuction shall be chosen [7]. Another indication for an inverse mini-abdominoplasty is a case when the downward traction asserted to the abdominal skin demonstrates an absence of sufficient laxity to bridge the gap of a full abdominoplasty. Whether a mini-abdominoplasty with floating umbilius or not is to be performed, depends on the vertical location of the umbilicus. If the umbilicus is proximal to the mid-level of the ksiphoid-pubis height, a floating umbilicus is indicated. If the umbilicus is between 1/2 and distal 1/3 of the vertical abdominal height, relocating the umbilicus further down should not be performed since it would distort the abdominal harmony [8] (Fig. 6.1).

It should be noted that performing mini-abdominoplasty without a full abdominal plication is a sure way to patient dissatisfaction. This is also valid for an incomplete plication covering only the lower part of the abdomen. In such a case, the tightening of the lower abdomen might even result in bulging of the upper abdomen.

The presence of substantial visceral fat accumulation prevents any successful result even if extensive muscular tightening would be performed. Such patients are contraindicated for any abdominal surgery, may it be liposuction or abdominoplasty, and are directed to dieticians or bariatric surgery centers.

Contraindications to mini-abdominoplasty are excessive skin and soft tissue in the upper abdomen, generalized laxity or soft-tissue excess of the entire abdominal wall, and patients presenting after massive weight loss.

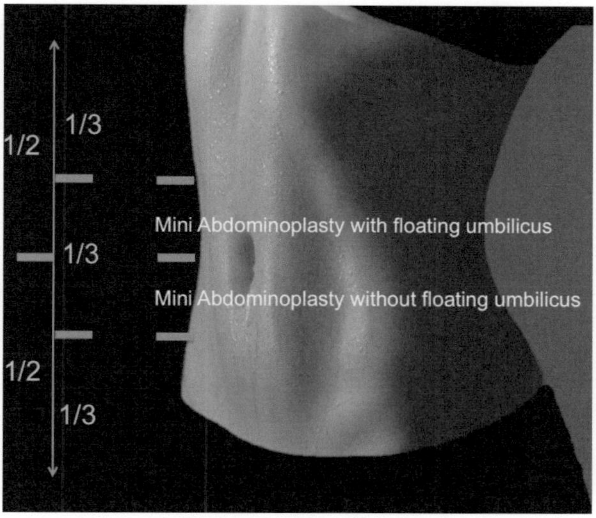

Fig. 6.1 If the umbilicus is vertically above the mid-level of the ksiphoid-pubis height a floating umbilicus is indicated. If the umbilicus is distally between 1/2 and 1/3 of ksiphoid-pubis height, a mini-abdominoplasty without a floating umbilicus is preferable, since moving the umbilicus further distally would distort the harmony of the abdomen. Usually a full abdominoplasty is performed if the umbilicus is distal to 2/3 of the abdominal height

Even though the candidates for mini-abdominoplasty are usually younger, healthier, and fitter than patients requiring more extensive procedures, any personal or family history of deep vein thrombosis (DVT) and/or pulmonary embolism (PE) is very important, and standard precautions should be taken due to the fact that like all forms of abdominoplasty this procedure also includes myofascial plication [9]. General precautions like cessation of smoking are important in all types of abdominoplasty procedures and should begin several weeks before and continue after the procedure [10–12].

Things to Remember

- Even though the candidates for mini-abdominoplasty are usually younger, healthier, and fitter, standard precautions should be taken due to the fact that, like all forms of abdominoplasty, this procedure also includes myofascial plication.
- The presence of substantial visceral fat accumulation prevents any successful result even if extensive muscular tightening would be performed. Such patients are contraindicated for any abdominal surgery.

6.3 Surgical Technique

6.3.1 Marking

Initially, preoperative photographs are taken in anterior, bent, right and left oblique, and right and left lateral views. Patients are marked in a standing position to delineate the areas for liposuction and skin incisions, wearing their preferred undergarments to confine the incision within the boundaries of her clothing.

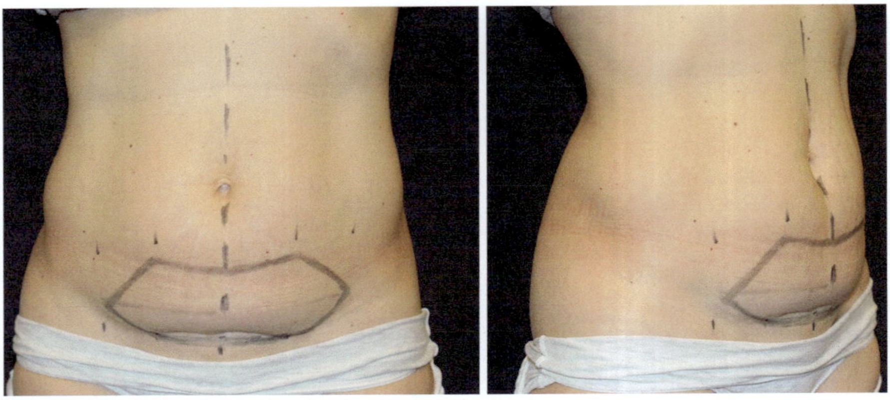

Fig. 6.2 A seagull shape is designed around 7–8 cm inferior to the umbilicus. This superior horizontal line is drawn gently upward, peaking up around 5–6 cm away on both sides, and then curving toward the lateral endings of the inferior incision line

Marking starts with a midline drawing from the xyphoid to the umbilicus and to the anterior vulvar commissure with the patient standing, which will serve also as a reference line to facilitate symmetry and to better appreciate any excess of tissue on either sides. Two paramedian vertical lines are also drawn 5–6 cm off the midline symmetrically.

Holding the skin excess in the lower abdomen, a curvilinear incision is marked in the natural inferior skinfold, extending in length slightly beyond the lateral skinfolds with the patient in a lateral hip-flexed position. A seagull shape superior line is designed around 7–8 cm inferior to the umbilicus. This superior horizontal line is drawn gently upward, peaking up around 5–6 cm away on both sides from the midline at the paramedian lines, and then curves downward toward the lateral endings of the inferior incision line. The amount of skin to be removed is double-checked by the surgeon grasping the skin and confirming that the upper and lower incisions meet (Fig. 6.2).

Simultaneously, the marking for the concurrent liposuction is drawn to address all areas of excess adiposity. This might include the entire abdomen, flanks, and mons pubis area. In inverse mini-abdominoplasty, the liposuction might be an important element in substantial majority of cases.

The definitive markings for the real amount of tissue resection are done on the operating table. The patients are dressed with thromboembolic deterrent stockings before they are called to the OR.

6.3.2 Positioning and Planning

Unless indicated otherwise, the surgery is usually performed under general anesthesia. In the OR, the operating table is checked to insure that it can be flexed prior to induction of anesthesia. The patient is placed in a supine position with silicone pillows under the knees to prevent nerve compressions during the surgery.

Afterward, the symmetry of the body and the arms is verified; a rolled towel of 5–10 cm in diameter is positioned behind the back of the patient at the level of the scapulae in order to decrease the unnatural backward leaning of the thorax, and the arms are loosely secured by wrapping them with gauze. A Foley catheter is inserted, sequential pneumatic compression devices are placed, and if indicated, anticoagulants are used.

To guarantee symmetry a 2-0 silk suture is placed in the midline at the level of the xyphoid. Vertical parallel lines to the midline at 5, 10, and 15 cm are drawn, and a symmetrical upper incision line with a seagull shape is obtained at the crossing of the vertical lines using the silk suture. The same drawing is performed for the planned lower incision.

If any liposuction is planned, it is performed immediately in the beginning of the abdominal procedure. The mini-abdominoplasty is done once the suction is completed (Fig. 6.3).

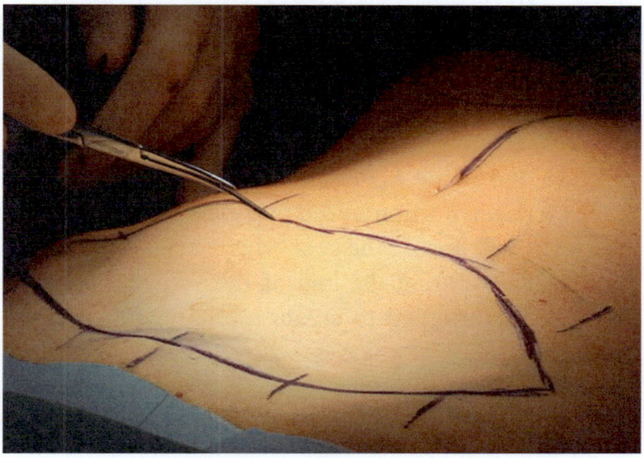

Fig. 6.3 To achieve symmetry a 2-0 silk suture is placed in the midline. Vertical parallel lines at 5, 10, and 15 cm are drawn, and a symmetrical upper incision line with a seagull shape is obtained at the crossing of the vertical lines using the silk suture. Afterward, the inferior incision line is drawn

Points to Remember

- The operating table is checked to ensure that it can be flexed prior to induction of anesthesia.
- A rolled towel is placed under the back at the level of each scapula bones to mimic natural standing position.
- Vertical parallel lines at 5, 10, and 15 cm are drawn, and a symmetrical upper incision line with a seagull shape is obtained at the crossing of the vertical lines using the silk suture. The same drawing is performed for the lower planned incision.

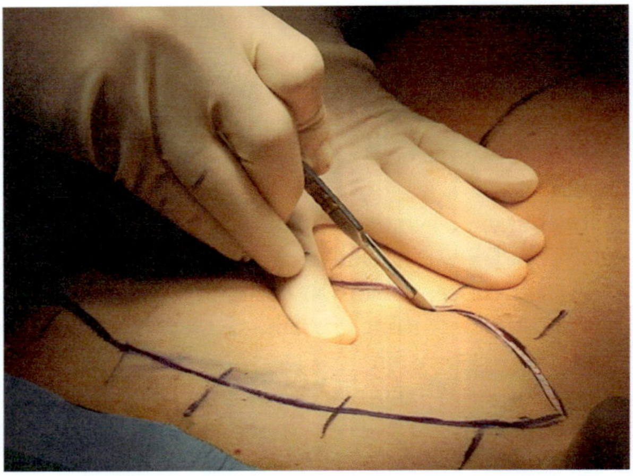

Fig. 6.4 A slightly beveled incision through the cutis is made through the superior seagull shape marking to achieve proper cutting angle, which will be beneficial for scar healing due to better suture line elevation

6.3.3 Incision and Upper Flap Elevation

First, the upper incision is made. A slightly beveled incision through the cutis is made through the superior seagull shape marking, while pulling the skin only downward in order to achieve proper cutting angle (Fig. 6.4).

Then, the blade bevels more to lie at 30° to the surface of the flap so the Scarpa's fascia portion of the flap is about 1 cm shorter than the skin portion. This maneuver will ensure the scar-edge elevation and an appropriate skin closure with good scar healing at the end of the surgery. The bilateral upward curves of the incision are designed to create a relative paramedian skin gap and median skin excess.

The supra and sub-scarpal fat is transversed until the surgeon reaches the abdominal wall. The large vessels are suture-ligated, and the rest of the dissection is done by electrocautery or harmonic scalpel, leaving the fine areolar tissue and their lymphatics over the fascia.

6.3.4 Floating Umbilicus

Once the umbilicus is reached, it is dissected from the surrounding tissue, a 2-0 Vicryl is placed at the base of the stalk to obliterate the base, and it is divided free from the abdominal wall just above the suture. Then, the dissection is continued up to the xyphoid resembling a narrow midline tunnel, sufficient to achieve rectus muscle repair and anterior sheath plication (Fig. 6.5a–f). If a mini-abdominoplasty without floating umbilicus is planned, the dissection is continued up to the ksiphoid using light retractors, without separating the umbilicus from the abdominal wall.

The lack of the lateral dissection will create a slight lateral tension at the closure of the skin. This, in conjunction with the initial paramedian skin gap due to the seagull incision, will help to narrow the waistline.

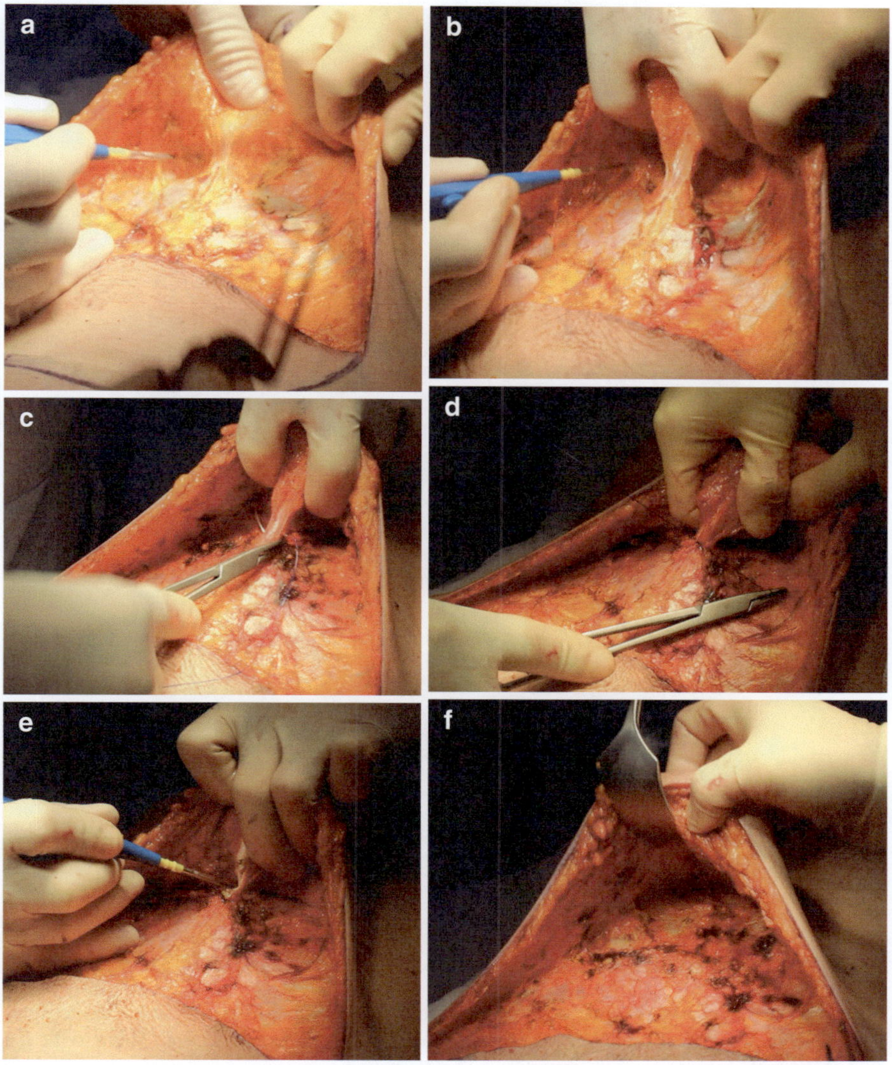

Fig. 6.5 (**a–f**) After the stalk is reached, a 2-0 Vicryl is placed at the base of the stalk, and it is divided free from the abdominal wall. Then the dissection is continued up to the xyphoid resembling a narrow midline tunnel, sufficient to achieve rectus muscle repair and anterior sheath plication

6.3.5 Lower Flap Elevation

Once the upper flap is elevated, a cold towel is placed into the dissected tunnel and around the flap in order to decrease capillary bleeding. The lower flap dissection is performed in the same way downward to the inguinal region (Fig. 6.6).

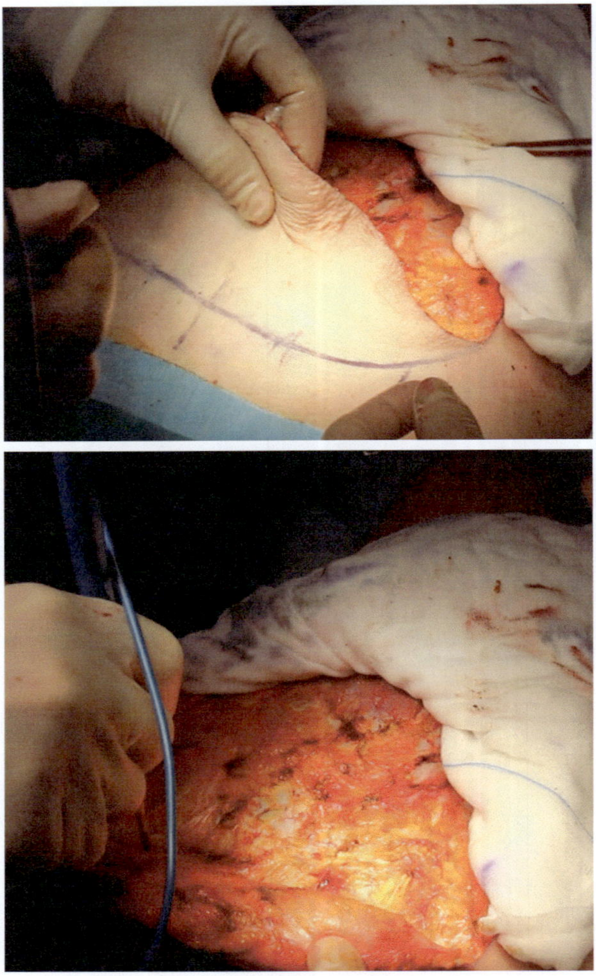

Fig. 6.6 The surgeon goes to the other side of the table according to his dominant hand (right-handed surgeons start on the *right side* of the table for the upper flap dissection, going to the *left side* of the table for inferior flap dissection). The dissection is continued few centimeters passing beyond the inferior marking

6.3.6 *Proximal Horizonto-vertical Plication*

It is important to note that the expansion of the abdomen due to the musculofascial laxity is a chronic three-dimensional deformation, i.e., tissue expansion, which happens in the horizontal plane as well as the vertical plane. A definitive treatment of this condition necessitates a Horizonto-vertical plication of the abdominal wall. The authors use spring sutures, a triple continuous over-and-over suture, which resembles a spring, or a helical coil, in order to tighten the fascia in horizontal as well as the vertical plane (Figs. 6.7 and 6.8).

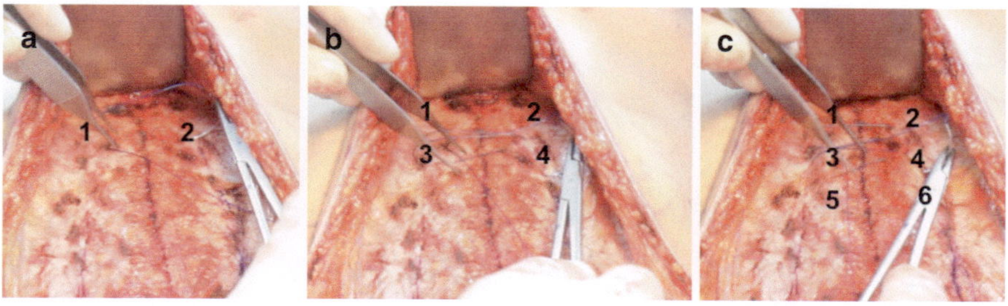

Fig. 6.7 (a–c)

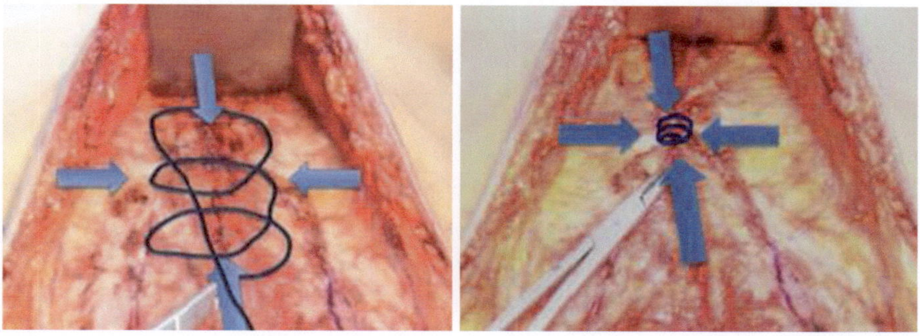

Fig. 6.8 The use of a triple continuous over-and-over spring sutures which resemble a helical coil, in order to tighten the fascia in the horizontal as well as the vertical plane

Starting from the upper end of the superior midline tunnel, a triple helix is created with 1-0 polypropylene. These buried sutures start with taking a bite at the left lateral edge of the diastasis, and then the right side, repeating three times to create a triple helical loop around the tread itself, fashioning a spring of Prolene. As the knot is tied, the fascia is fastened in the horizontal as well as the vertical plane. These separate triple helical spring sutures are used as many as needed till the surgeon comes to the level of the stalk.

Since a mini-abdominoplasty with an incomplete plication covering only the lower part of the abdomen usually results in further bulging of the upper abdomen, the authors advise to perform full-length plication of the midline, even with patients who initially do not have severe upper abdominal complaints.

6.3.7 *Relocation and Anchoring of the Umbilicus*

Once the plication reaches the original umbilical stalk level, the amount of umbilical relocation is calculated. The stalk is re-anchored usually 3–4 cm inferior to its original vertical level.

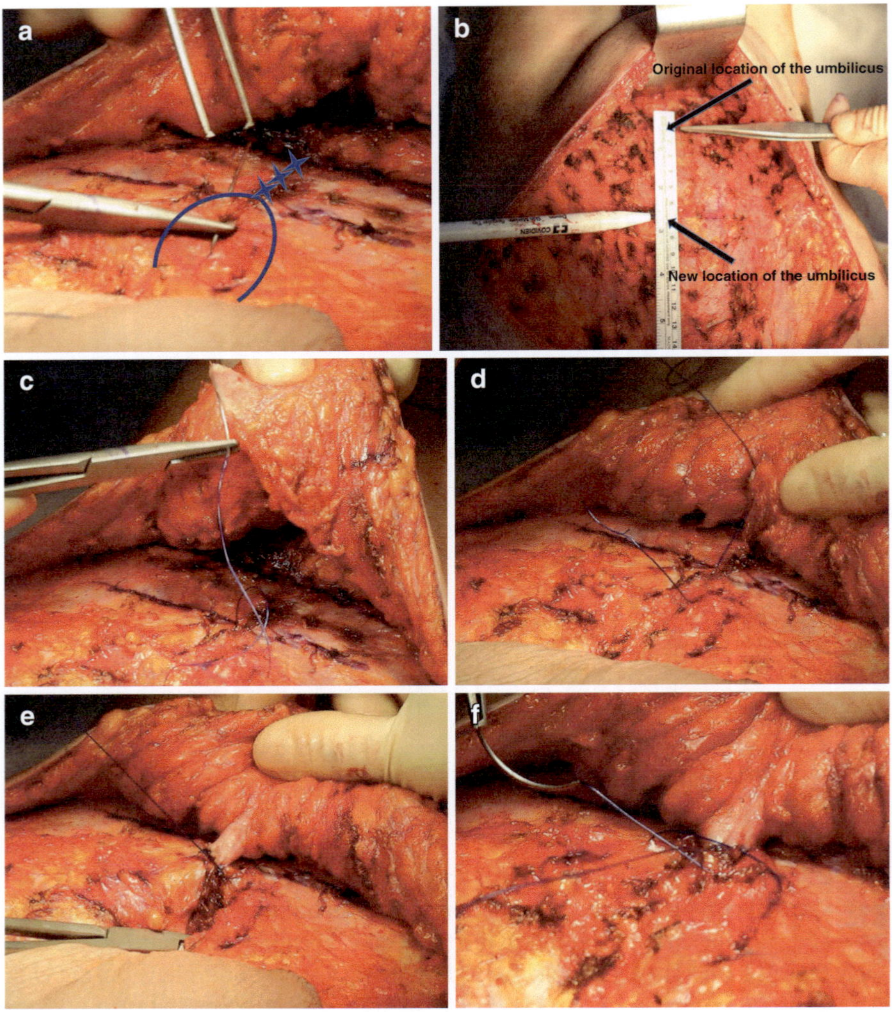

Fig. 6.9 (**a**–**f**) The plication is continued using the helical spring sutures down to the planned level of the new umbilicus location, which is usually few centimeters caudal to the original location. Three 2-0 Vicryl sutures are placed between the umbilical stalk and the semi-buried abdominal wall fascia at the midline

First, the fascia is plicated further to the new umbilical attachment level, and three 2-0 Vicryl sutures are placed between the base of the stalk and the midline of the abdominal wall, which is already semi-buried at 3, 6, and 9 o'clock (Fig. 6.9a–f).

Umbilical re-anchoring has many advantages, including the following:

- Improved tightening of the epigastric skin, avoiding residual bulging.
- Decreased tension on the hypogastrium.
- Re-balancing the abdominal aesthetics in patients with long upper torso.
- The created upper abdominal tension will divide the median skin into two skinfolds, thus fashioning the double-rectus fold illusion.

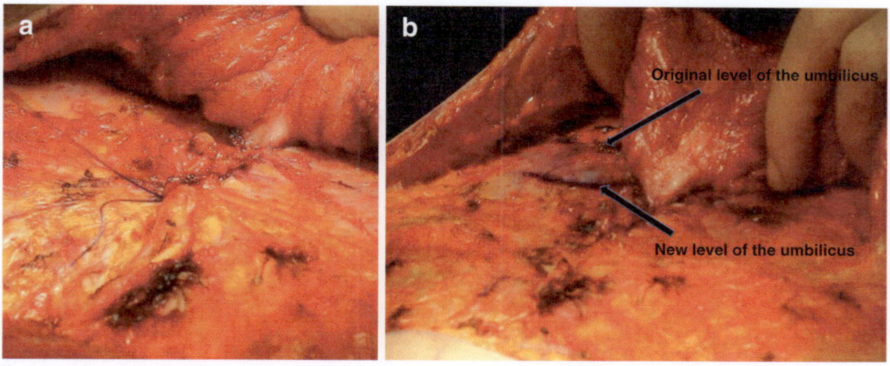

Fig. 6.10 (**a**, **b**) Once the stalk is securely re-anchored to the new position, the plication is continued, thus pulling the base of the stalk deep into the plicated midline portion of the abdominal wall

6.3.8 Caudal Plication

After the stalk is sutured to the abdominal fascia, the plication is continued downward and completed. Hence, the attached stalk base is automatically pulled inward and buried deep with the inverted fascia, creating the natural umbilical depression.

The 4–5-cm shift of the umbilicus from the original to its new location will be clearly recognizable and helps dealing with the skin problems and striae immediately above the navel (Fig. 6.10a, b).

6.3.9 Fascial Anesthesia

Meticulous hemostasis is ensured after the plication. About 40 cc of 0.25 % bupivacaine solution is prepared, and around 10 cc of this solution is injected per quadrant just beneath the external fascia of the rectus and the external oblique muscles with blunt needles to anesthetize the regional nerves to the abdominal muscles. The trajectory of the needle should be visualized by translucency through the fascia to ensure the proper depth of the injection [13]. This local anesthetic injection immensely decreases the patient's need for narcotics for the whole postoperative period (Fig. 6.11).

6.3.10 Skin Excision and Closure

Resection of the mini-abdominoplasty flap is done after the umbilicus is secured to its new location. If there is a necessity, the preoperative markings are realigned according to the skin excess and the inferior skin flap is resected (Fig. 6.12). After the excision is done, a final inspection for hemostasis is performed prior to the

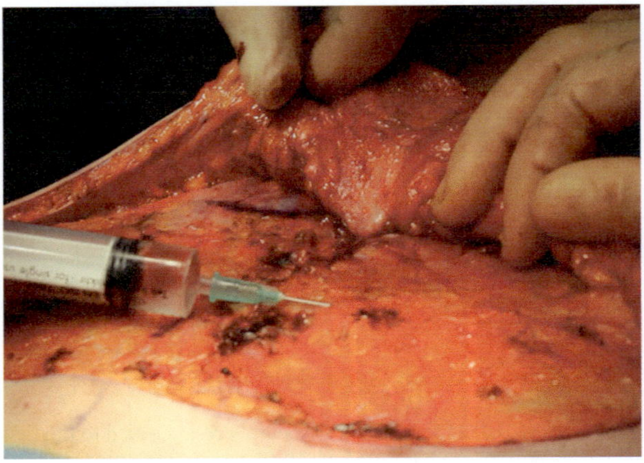

Fig. 6.11 Ten cc of local aesthetic solution is injected per quadrant just beneath the external fascia of the rectus and the external oblique muscles with blunt needles to anesthetize the regional nerves to the abdominal muscles. The trajectory of the needle should be visualized by translucency through the fascia to ensure the proper depth of the injection

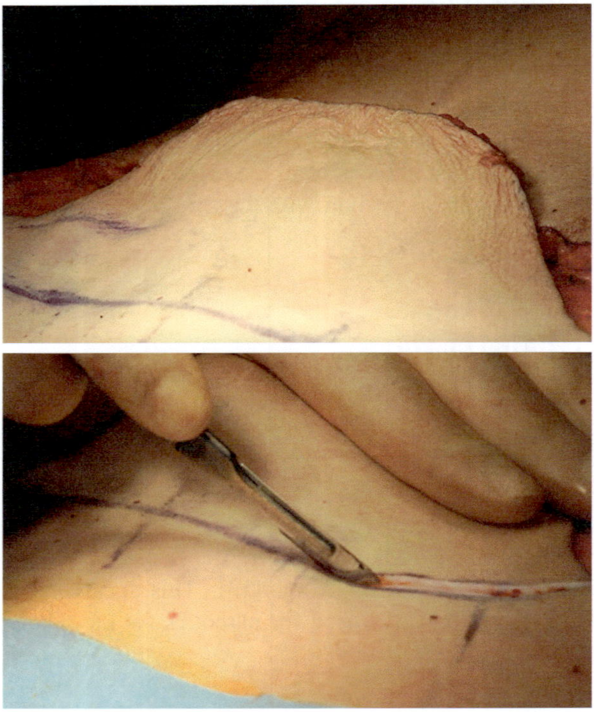

Fig. 6.12 Resection of the skin excess is done after the umbilicus is secured to its new location. The superior flap edge is pulled down below the inferior flap, and the preoperative marking is verified. If there is a necessity, the marking is realigned according to the skin excess, and the inferior skin flap is resected with careful hemostasis of edges

closure. Once the hemostasis is ensured, the realignment of the superior and inferior flaps is planned.

In order to prevent the incision line to drift upward, a symmetrical marking is done on the abdominal wall where both flaps are going to be secured. Securing the flaps to this line will ensure symmetry as well as the stability of the scar height.

Since the upper flap has a tendency to drift laterally and also the incision line is longer than the inferior flap edge, there is a need to pull the superior flap medially and shorten the incision length. This is obtained by marking the vertical closure lines differently on both flaps. At the upper flap edge, 5th and 4th centimeters and on the lower edge, 4th and 3rd centimeters are marked symmetrically from the midline (Fig. 6.13) advancing superior flap inferomedially. Scarpa's fascia is approximated and fixed to the abdominal wall at the level of the previous marking, thus ensuring the symmetry of the scar as well as preventing the superior drifting using 2-0 Vicryl sutures. These sutures also take the tension off of the skin closure and allow for fine skin closure. At the same time, the upper incision is shortened symmetrically fitting the lower incision, and the upper flap ends are pulled medially.

For the final closure, two 3-0 bidirectional barbed sutures are used in the superficial fat layer and the dermis on either side of the midline in a running fashion.

Two multi-perforated drains are placed beneath the abdominal flap in a crisscross fashion to avoid kinking, exiting in the pubic skin without any fixation. The incision line is steri-stripped, and horizontal splinting tape dressings are placed around the abdomen followed by an elastic girdle (Fig. 6.14).

Things to Remember

- A slightly beveled incision through the cutis is made through the superior seagull shape marking to achieve proper cutting angle, which will be beneficial for scar healing due to better suture line elevation.
- Performing mini-abdominoplasty without a full abdominal plication is a sure way to patient dissatisfaction. This is also valid for an incomplete plication covering only the lower part of the abdomen. In such a case, the tightening of the lower abdomen might even result in worsening of the upper abdominal bulging.
- Umbilical re-anchoring has many advantages, including improved tightening of the epigastric skin, decreased tension on the hypogastrium, rebalancing the abdominal aesthetics in patients with long upper torso, and fashioning the double-rectus fold illusion.
- The subfascial local anesthetic injection immensely decreases the patient's need for narcotics for the "whole" postoperative period.
- In order to prevent the incision line to drift upward, a symmetrical marking is done on the abdominal wall where both flaps are going to be secured. Securing the flaps to this line will ensure symmetry as well as the stability of the scar height.

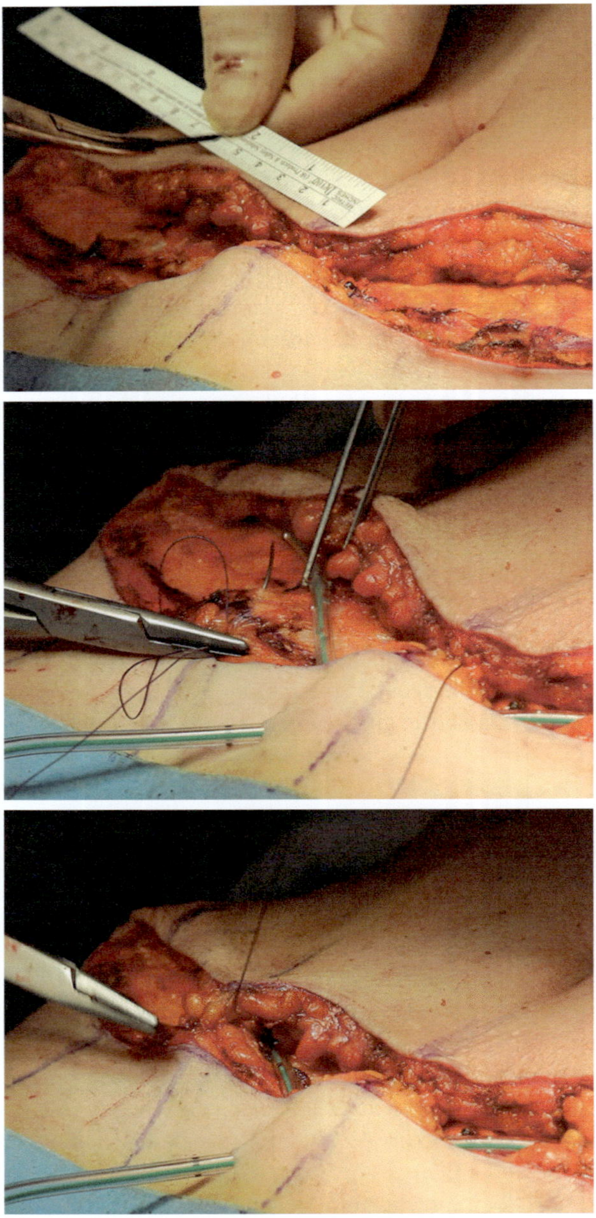

Fig. 6.13 Since the upper incision line is longer than the inferior flap edge, there is a need to pull the superior flap medially and also shorten the incision length. This is obtained by marking the vertical closure lines differently on both flaps. At the upper flap edge, 5th and 4th centimeters and on the lower edge, 4th and 3rd centimeters are marked symmetrically from the midline. Suturing these vertical marks together will shorten the upper incision symmetrically fitting the lower incision, and the upper flap ends are pulled medially

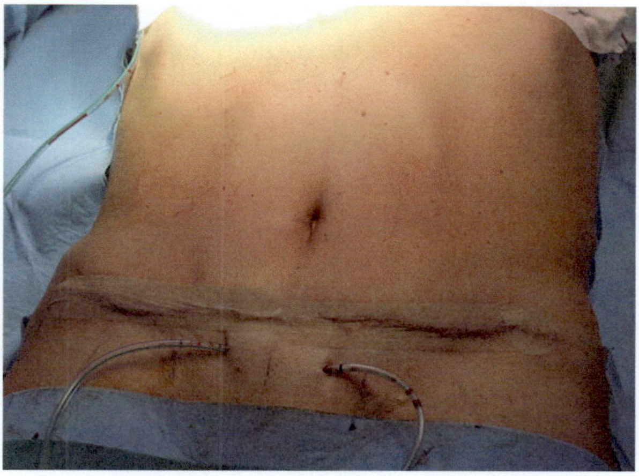

Fig. 6.14 Final closure: two 3-0 bidirectional barbed sutures are used in the superficial fat layer and the dermis on either side of the midline in a running fashion. Two multi-perforated drains are placed beneath the abdominal flap in a crisscross fashion to avoid kinking, exiting in the pubic skin without any fixation

6.3.11 Postoperative Care

It is important to keep in mind that a full abdominal plication shall be performed also in mini-abdominoplasty, which ensures a satisfactory outcome but necessitates a proper postoperative care. At the end of the procedure, the patient is warmed with a warming blanket and monitored in the recovery room until the patient becomes stable. Here an elastic compressive binder is applied and worn continuously for at least 2 weeks. The patients are given intravenous fluids and antibiotics for the first postoperative day. A clear liquid diet is started the same day, and the diet is advanced gradually as tolerated. Supportive stockings and pneumatic boots are used until the patient is walking [14].

The patient is encouraged to be in a semi-sitting position the night after surgery with immediate and progressive ambulation in a semi-flexed position. The drains are removed when the drainage declines to less than 30 cc per 24 h, usually the next day. After the drains are removed, the patient is sent home on the first day of the surgery.

The patients are discharged from the hospital with oral antibiotics and anti-inflammatory medication. The first follow-up visit is at the 48 h, where all the splinting tapes are removed and the patient is encouraged to take full shower.

Full activity for daily life is resumed in 2–3 weeks after surgery. The patients are allowed to perform cardio training after 4 weeks, but abdominal workout is prohibited for 3 months (Figs. 6.15, 6.16, and 6.17).

Box: Postoperative Instructions for Mini-abdominoplasty

- Use the incentive spirometer.
- Avoid smoking or exposure to nicotine-containing products.
- Drink plenty of fluids: 2 l/day is the goal.
- Move legs frequently while resting and walk regularly.
- Continue to take medications as instructed.
- Maintain a slightly flexed position at the waist for the first 1 week.
- Wear the abdominal binder for 3 weeks at all times except for showering.
- Shower on the second day after the first visit.
- Steri-strips are taken away on the first-week visit.
- No driving for 1 week.
- Easy walking after 2 weeks.
- No vigorous activity for 3 weeks.
- No abdominal training for 3 months.

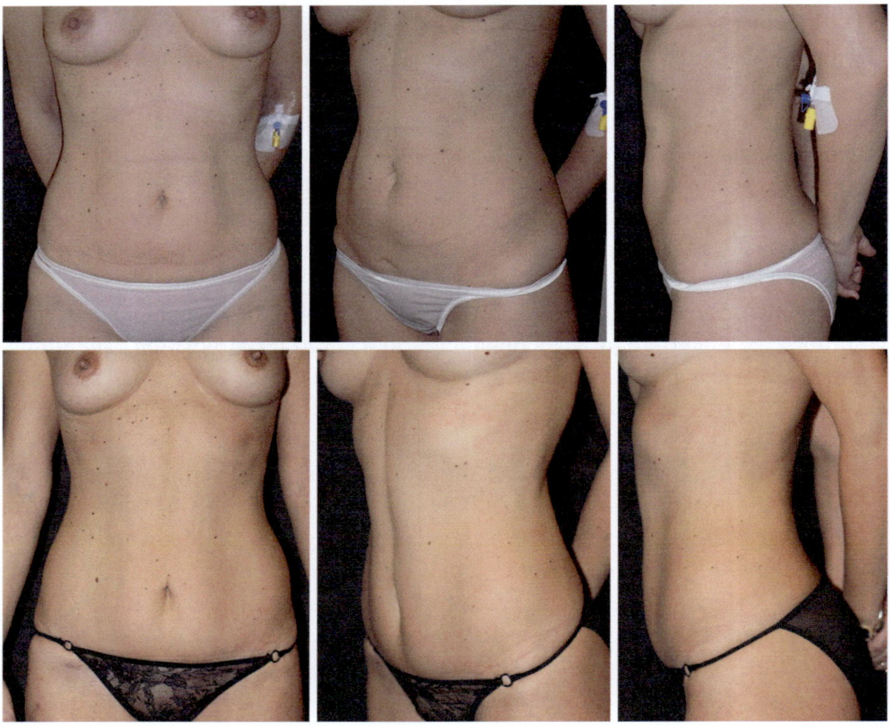

Fig. 6.15 A 47-year-old woman. This patient demonstrated good skin quality, poor waistline definition, and contour secondary to abdominal wall laxity without any significant adiposity. After inverse mini-abdominoplasty with full-length horizontovertical myofascial plication without any concurrent liposuction, the patient demonstrates dramatically improved abdominal contour, waistline, and silhouette, with false rectus folds

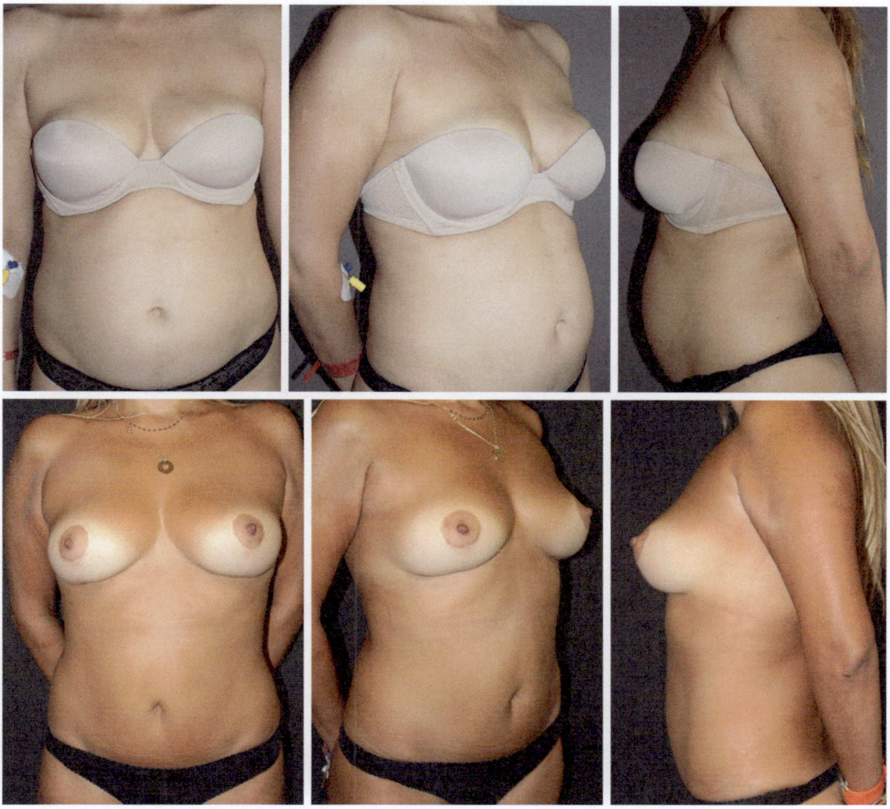

Fig. 6.16 A 49-year-old woman. This patient demonstrated moderate skin quality, poor waistline definition, and bulging abdomen secondary to abdominal wall laxity and moderate adiposity. After inverse mini-abdominoplasty with full-length horizontovertical myofascial plication with minimal liposuction limited to posterior waist, she demonstrates dramatically reduced abdominal bulging, improved silhouette, and moderate false rectus folds

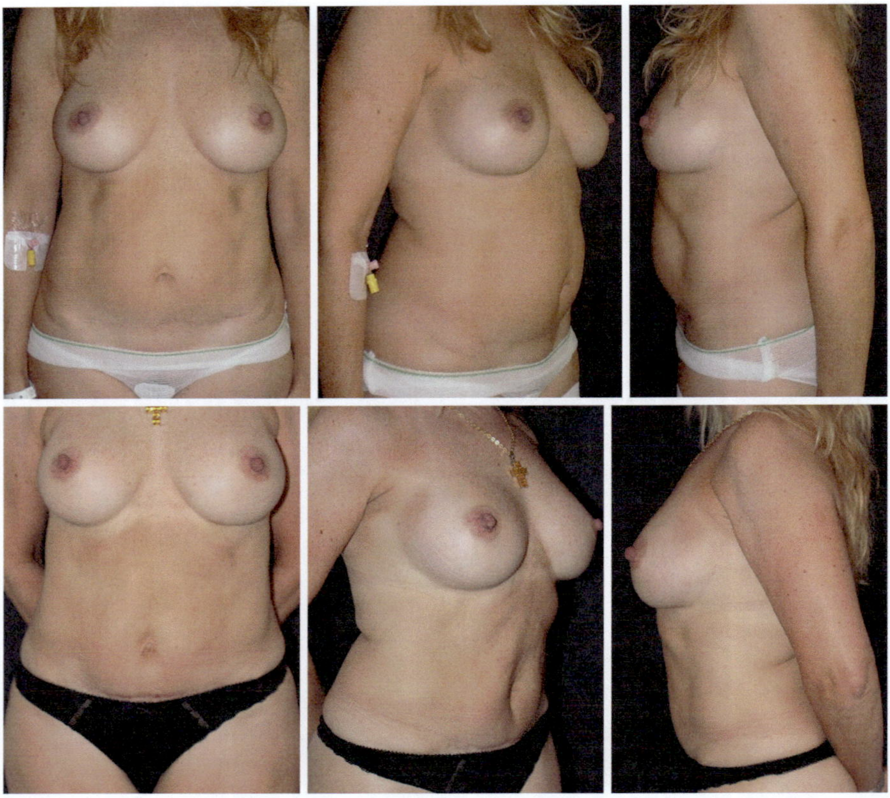

Fig. 6.17 A 56-year-old woman. This patient demonstrated moderate skin quality, poor waist contour secondary to abdominal wall laxity, and moderate adiposity. After inverse mini-abdominoplasty with full-length horizontovertical myofascial plication without any concurrent liposuction, the patient demonstrates improved abdominal contour, waistline, and silhouette, with false rectus folds

References

1. Sozer SO, Agullo FJ, Santillan AA, Wolf C. Decision making in abdominoplasty. Aesthetic Plast Surg. 2007;31(2):117–27.
2. Hunstad JP, Repta R. Atlas of abdominoplasty. Philadelphia: Saunders/Elsevier; 2009. p. 33–45.
3. Shiffman MA, Mirrafati S. Aesthetic surgery of the abdominal wall. Berlin/New York: Springer; 2005. p. 87–93.
4. Greminger RF. The mini-abdominoplasty. Plast Reconstr Surg. 1987;79:356–64.
5. Wilkerson TS, Swartz BE. Individual modifications in body contour surgery: the "limited" abdominoplasty. Plast Reconstr Surg. 1986;77:779–83.
6. Mast BA, Hurwitz DJ. Mini-abdominoplasty. Operative Tech Plast Reconstr Surg. 1996;3:38.
7. Shestak KC. Marriage abdominoplasty expands the mini-abdominoplasty concept. Plast Reconstr Surg. 1999;103:1020–31.

8. Hoyos AE, Perez ME, Castillo L, Dynamic definition mini-lipoabdominoplasty combining multilayer liposculpture, fat grafting and muscular plication. Aesthet Surg J. 2013;33(4):545–60.
9. McDevitt NB. Deep vein thrombosis prophylaxis. American society of plastic and reconstructive surgeons. Plast Reconstruct Surg. 1999;104:1923. Davison SP, Venturi ML, Attinger CE et al. Prevention of venous thromboembolism in the plastic surgery patient. Plast Reconstruct Surg. 2004;114:43.
10. Krueger JK, Rohrich RJ. Clearing the smoke: the scientific rationale for tobacco abstention with plastic surgery. Plast Reconstr Surg. 2001;15:108–1063.
11. Manassa EH, Hertl CH, Olbrisch RR. Wound healing problems in smokers and nonsmokers after 132 abdominoplasties. Plast Reconstr Surg. 2003;111:2082.
12. Matarasso A. Classification and patient selection in abdominoplasty. Oper Tech Plast Reconstr Surg. 1996;3:7–14.
13. Matarasso A. Traditional abdominoplasty. Clin Plast Surg. 2010;37(3):415–37.
14. Shiffman MA, Mirrafati S. Aesthetic surgery of the abdominal wall. Berlin/New York: Springer; 2005. p. 115–20. ISBN 978-3-540-27263-2.

Chapter 7
Abdominoplasty as a Combined Procedure

Derya Ozçelik and Renato Saltz

7.1 Statistics

Abdominoplasty is one of the most requested aesthetic procedures because of the immediate improvement it can produce in a patient's body contour. According to the American Society for Aesthetic Plastic Surgery (ASAPS), it is currently the third most common cosmetic surgical procedure performed in the United States, with 180,717 procedures (172,634 women, 8,083 men) performed in 2015 [1]. The massive increase in weight loss procedures being performed, with a 16-fold increase in the past decade [1–4], significantly contributed to the increase in the number of abdominoplasties.

Abdominoplasty is usually performed as a combined operation with other aesthetic procedures. Frequently, female patients who are unhappy with the appearance of their abdomen are also displeased with the shape or size of their breasts. Following pregnancy, abdominoplasty and aesthetic breast surgery performed in one operation is even called with a special name "the mommy makeover" by the popular media. Although it is commonly presumed that the rate of combined procedures with abdominoplasty is increasing steadily with the "makeover" concept [5, 6], latest data indicate that this is not the case. Winocour et al. reported that between 2008 and 2013, the rate of combined procedures dropped from 67.6 % to 65.5 % ($p<0.01$) [7]. In the same study, Winocour et al. analyzed the patients who underwent abdominoplasty between 2008 and 2013 from the CosmetAssure database. The authors identified 25,478 abdominoplasties from 183,914 procedures in the database. Of these,

D. Ozçelik, MD (✉)
Plastic Reconstructive and Aesthetic Surgery Department, Sakarya University Medical Faculty, Sakarya, Turkey
e-mail: deryaozcelik34@gmail.com

R. Saltz
Plastic Reconstructive and Aesthetic Surgery Department, Saltz Plastic Surgery and Spa Vitória, Salt Lake City and Park City, UT, USA
e-mail: rsaltz@saltzplasticsurgery.com

K.T. Tiryaki (ed.), *Inverse Abdominoplasty*, DOI 10.1007/978-3-319-39310-0_7

8975 patients (35.2 %) had abdominoplasty alone, and 16,503 (64.8 %) underwent additional procedures. In other words, abdominoplasty was reported in combination with other procedures in two-thirds of the patients. In the same series, it was reported that this result was in contrast to other non-abdominoplasty cosmetic procedures, where only 24.5 % of patients underwent combined procedures. From 2008 to 2013, although there was a steady increase in the overall number of abdominoplasties performed, the percentage of patients undergoing combined abdominoplasty procedures remained stable (67.6–65.5 %, respectively) [7]. Interestingly, in an article published in 1973 including a small series of 44 cases, abdominoplasty was also reported to be combined with other surgeries in two-thirds of patients [8].

Winocour et al. reported that among 16,503 patients having combined procedure with abdominoplasty, the most commonly performed aesthetic procedure in combination with abdominoplasty was liposuction (42 %), followed by aesthetic breast surgery (26 %) (i.e., augmentation, reduction, revision of breast implant procedures, mastopexy, male breast surgery), and liposuction plus aesthetic breast surgery (20 %) [7]. The other procedures combined with abdominoplasty include body procedures (i.e., brachioplasty, buttock lift, calf implant, labioplasty, lower body lift, thigh lift, upper body lift) and/or face procedures (i.e., blepharoplasty, brow lift, cheek implant, chin augmentation, face lift, facial resurfacing, hair replacement, otoplasty, rhinoplasty).

Things to Remember

- Abdominoplasty is combined with other procedures in *two-thirds of the patients*.
- The most commonly performed procedure in combination with abdominoplasty is *liposuction*, followed by *aesthetic breast surgery*.

7.2 Preoperative Preparation of Abdominoplasty as a Combined Procedure

In the decision to perform a combined procedure with abdominoplasty, patient selection is of significant consequence. Prior to any elective surgery, the surgeon should confirm that no preexisting health conditions preclude lengthy general anesthesia. Preoperative laboratory work would be prudent prior to a multi-region combined procedure. In cases of prior cardiac or pulmonary conditions, appropriate specialists should be consulted in addition to the anesthesiologist. The surgeon should also provide an honest estimate of the total length of the combined procedure depending on prior surgical experience and availability of appropriate assistants. The concept of a “surgical team” familiar with combined body contouring procedures and the importance of “time efficiency” cannot be overemphasized in these types of cases. According to American Society of Plastic Surgeons (ASPS) Patient Safety Committee guidelines, elective surgery should ideally be limited to no more than 6 hours.

Patients should be weight stable for several months and nutritionally stable prior to surgery. While a normal body mass index (BMI) is not always a realistic goal, an obese patient should be counseled on further weight loss prior to surgery, as they are not likely to derive optimal results from surgery.

Preoperative evaluation should focus on both personal and family history of coagulopathy, including a history of multiple miscarriages. Smokers should not undergo abdominoplasty or combined procedures due to high likelihoods of wound complication and pulmonary compromise. Oral contraceptives and hormone replacement therapies can increase thrombotic risk and should be stopped weeks prior to surgery.

In the combined procedure population, the patient's dedication to total body transformation is extremely high, and the expectation no less so. The outcome of the surgery is expected to be transformative and staggering given the monetary and time commitment of the patient. It is imperative that extensive preoperative discussions occur using the patient's own photographs outlining the realistic goals of surgery. When sharing photographs from prior surgeries, the representative photographs should be close in age and body habitus to the patient. The limits of patient's own anatomy due to natural body shape, age, skin quality, and prior surgical scars should be carefully outlined. The patient should also be informed that in any aesthetic surgery, there is always room for improvement and revision further down the line.

Things to Remember

- Patients should be *weight stable* for several months and *nutritionally stable* prior to abdominoplasty surgery.
- *Patients treated with abdominoplasty alone* typically have *lower BMIs* than *patients undergoing lipoabdominoplasty*.

7.3 Discussion About the Safety of Abdominoplasty Combinations

When combining other aesthetic procedures with abdominoplasty, careful consideration is essential at all stages of the process, including patient selection, preoperative planning, intraoperative technique, and postoperative regimen. Combination of procedures has the presumed benefit of requiring a single anesthetic, reduced overall recovery period, and reduced costs [9, 10]. Ultimately, the feasibility of combining abdominoplasty with other procedures rests on the requirement that the entire operation must be as safe as each of its component procedures if performed individually—without compromising the quality of each individual procedure. That is to say, when abdominoplasty is performed in conjunction with other aesthetic procedures, there should not be an increase in abdominoplasty-related complications such as seroma, hematoma, wound dehiscence, or tissue necrosis. Any presumed advantage must be weighed against the potential for adverse events [11, 12].

In literature, there is still an ongoing discussion about the complication rate of the abdominoplasty and abdominoplasty-combined procedures because of uneven profile of the patients like different BMIs.

Winocour et al. [7] evaluated 25,478 abdominoplasties (8975 patients (35.2 %) had abdominoplasty alone and 16,503 patients (64.8 %) underwent additional procedures) to evaluate significant risk factors associated with complications and to compare complication rates of different procedure combinations in a large, prospective, multicenter database. It was reported that significant risk factors ($p<0.05$) included male sex (relative risk versus female sex, 1.8), age 55 years or older (relative risk versus age 55 years or younger, 1.4), body mass index greater than or equal to 30 (relative risk versus BMI less than or equal to 30, 1.3), multiple procedures (relative risk versus single procedure, 1.5), and procedure performance in a hospital or surgical center versus office-based surgical suite (relative risk, 1.6). Among 25,478 abdominoplasty cases, the number of complications recorded was 1012 (4.0 % overall rate versus 1.4 % in other aesthetic surgery procedures). The most common complications seen with abdominoplasty were hematoma (1.3 percent), infection (1.1 percent), suspected or confirmed venous thromboembolism (0.8 percent), and pulmonary dysfunction (0.3 percent). This had a similar distribution to other cosmetic procedures. When specific procedure combinations were analyzed, there was significant variation in the complication rate: abdominoplasty alone, 3.1 %; abdominoplasty combined with liposuction, 3.8 %; abdominoplasty combined with a breast procedure, 4.3 %; abdominoplasty combined with liposuction and a breast procedure, 4.6 %; abdominoplasty combined with a body-contouring procedure, 6.8 %; abdominoplasty combined with liposuction and a body-contouring procedure, 10.4 %. Combining liposuction with abdominoplasty also increased the risk of possible or confirmed venous thromboembolism from 0.5 % to 1.1 % ($p<0.05$). They [7] concluded that abdominoplasty is associated with a higher complication rate compared with other aesthetic procedures. Combined procedures can significantly increase complication rates and should be considered carefully in higher risk patients.

Saad et al. conducted a retrospective longitudinal analysis between 2005 and 2010 using California Office of Statewide Health Planning and Development Ambulatory Surgery Database [13]. Patients were included if they had undergone an abdominoplasty or any other procedures that was identified as frequently performed concurrently with abdominoplasty. Patients' subsequent inpatient admissions and emergency department visits were identified. Outcomes analyzed were the 30-day and 1-year venous thromboembolism rates, 30-day hospital admission rate, 30-day emergency department visit rate, and 30-day mortality rate. At result, a total of 477,741 patients were analyzed of whom 16,893 had undergone two concurrent procedures. The 12-month venous thromboembolism rate was 0.57 % for patients undergoing abdominoplasty, 0.20 % for liposuction, 0.12 % for breast procedures, 0.32 % for hernia repair, 0.28 % for face procedures, and 0.28 % for thigh lift/brachioplasty. Greater than additive 30-day and 1-year venous thromboembolism rates were observed among patients who underwent an abdominoplasty and liposuction (0.68–0.81 %, respectively) and those who underwent an abdominoplasty and hernia repair (0.93 %). In conclusion, they thought that some combinations of elective outpatient procedures conferred an additive and sometimes more than additive venous thromboembolism risk [13].

On the other hand, for the study results of Saad et al., Swanson [14] made a different comment as follows:

'Saad et al. [13] concluded that combining abdominoplasty and liposuction or hernia repair created an increased risk of venous thromboembolism that was greater than additive. Saad et al. [13] define statistical significance as $p<0.05$. It is not clear from the authors' statistical description how they determined p values for comparing expected and observed complication rates. The additive rate of venous thromboembolism within 1 year of combined lipoabdominoplasty is 0.77 % (0.57 + 0.20 %); the observed rate was 0.81 %. This difference is so small that subtracting just one affected patient ($n=23$ rather than $n=24$) would make the rates identical. The expected rate for abdominoplasty combined with hernia repair (0.57 + 0.32 % = 0.89 %) could not be closer to the observed rate (0.93 %). Adding or subtracting a single affected patient would make the difference between rates greater. Nevertheless, the authors cite a trend toward statistical significance that they are confident would be "further augmented with a larger sample size." It should be noted that a comparison of a calculation representing the sum of the incidences of venous thromboembolism for the individual procedures versus the observed incidence of venous thromboembolism after lipoabdominoplasty does not lend itself to a statistically valid test that could produce a reliable p value in the first place.'

Additionally, patients' characteristics are very important to make a healthy comparison between the procedures and their complication rates. Among them, body mass index is an important confounding variable. Patients treated with abdominoplasty alone typically have lower body mass indices than patients undergoing lipoabdominoplasty [15, 16]. Saad et al. [13] recognized that obesity is a risk factor for venous thromboembolism [17]. Body mass index may be controlled using an analysis of covariance [18]. The actual volume of liposuction aspirate that can be safely removed during a combined procedure is also important and as yet unknown. Therefore, restricting liposuction in combined procedures is the topic of many other debates.

On the other hand, Hester et al. [17] did not, in fact, find a significantly increased risk of venous thromboembolism when combining abdominoplasty and liposuction as claimed [13]. On the contrary, these investigators [17] concluded that obesity represented the only significant risk factor not procedural complexity. Soltani et al. [19] reported a venous thromboembolism risk of 0.06 % after abdominoplasty alone versus 0.07 % when abdominoplasty was combined with one other procedure, 0.08 % when combined with two other procedures, but did not suggest that these tiny differences were statistically significant or greater than additive as claimed [13]. Umbilical and ventral hernias are often repaired at the time of rectus plication. The suggestion that such a repair "intensifies the insult on the venous system" [13] is still contraversial.

Performing abdominoplasty in a combined body contouring procedure has the potential for increased postoperative pain limiting early ambulation as well as the theoretical potential for increased incidence of thrombophilia owing to the length of the procedure and prolonged immobilization. In the event of a complication after a combination of procedures, the surgeon might be unfairly blamed for "doing too much surgery at one time." Actually, with optimal patient selection and preoperative planning, modern abdominoplasty can be safely combined with other aesthetic procedures. With cautious preoperative workup and limiting the number of hours under general anesthesia, combined procedures parlay the potential benefits of single anesthesia, decreased total recovery time, and decreased expense to the patient. For decades now, plastic surgeons have been safely combining liposuction with abdominoplasty [15, 16]. Approximately two-thirds of abdominoplasties are performed with other procedures [19]. Lipoabdominoplasty produces higher levels of patient satisfaction and greater improvement of quality of life than either liposuction or abdominoplasty alone and avoids a second operation [15].

Things to Remember

- For abdominoplasty; significant *risk factors: male sex, age ≥55 years, BMI ≥ 30, combined surgery.*
- It is widely held that *obesity* is an independent risk factor for systemic morbidity like venous thromboembolism and local wound healing complications.
- *Combining liposuction with abdominoplasty increases the risk of venous thromboembolism.*

  Winocour et al.: Combining liposuction with abdominoplasty increases the risk of possible or confirmed venous thromboembolism from 0.5 % to 1.1 %

  Saad et al.: Combining liposuction with abdominoplasty increases the risk of venous thromboembolism within 12-month from 0.57 % to 0.8 %

  Soltani et al.: Combining one other procedure with abdominoplasty increases the risk of venous thromboembolism from 0.06 % to 0.07 %

7.4 Abdominoplasty Combined with Liposuction

As combined procedure with abdominoplasty, important contributions from Illouz [20] with his "mesh undermining" by performing liposuction of the abdomen and then "end block" removal of all infraumbilical tissue in selected patients started a new era in abdominoplasty. Matarasso [21, 22] described the treatment of different abdominal regions with major and minor risks of liposuction at the same time of the abdominoplasty. Saldanha [23, 24] combined many of these innovative and provocative techniques with his stellar contribution called as *lipoabdominoplasty* where liposuction of the abdomen was combined to rectus muscle plication through selective and safe undermining of the abdominal flap in the supraumbilical area by preserving the lateral rectus muscle perforators, thus increasing blood supply to the abdominal flap and its survival, decreasing the incidence of seroma and other complications of traditional abdominoplasty.

We and others have described the concept of abdominoplasty combined with liposuction for flap suctioning or contouring of adjacent areas. Principles of perioperative decision-making and intraoperative technical details to ensure synergistic aesthetic benefits from this combination have been addressed and are continuing to evolve [21, 22, 25, 26]. The potential advantages of abdominoplasty with concurrent liposuction (lipoabdominoplasty) include a better postoperative cosmetic result and a possible reduction in the need for revision surgery (Figs. 7.1 and 7.2).

Ousterhout demonstrated the feasibility of combining abdominoplasty and high-volume suction lipectomy in the obese patient [27], and Dillerud showed that neither obesity nor liposuction increased flap necrosis in abdominoplasty [28]. It is widely held, however, that obesity is an independent risk factor for local wound healing complications and systemic morbidity [29–31].

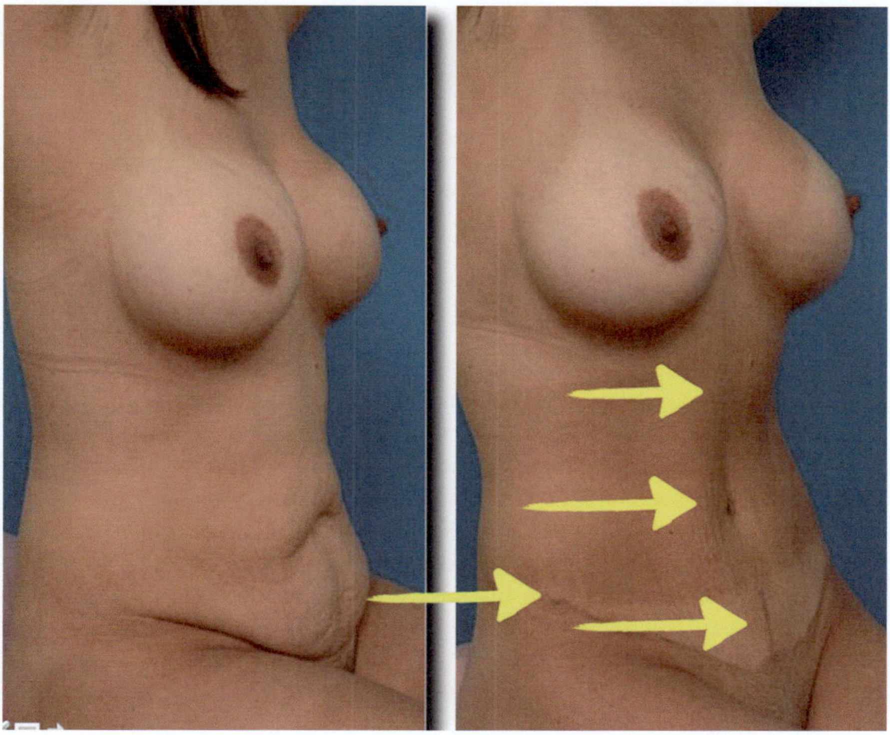

Fig. 7.1 (Slide 2 in PPT) – before and after "sit-down position" after combined procedure – abdominoplasty, liposuction of the back and flanks, implant exchange, and capsulotomies. *Arrows* from top to bottom, outline the supraumbilical midline sulcus, a small "mysterious" umbilicus, the length of the lower abdominal scar are determined by the location and length of the most lateral skinfold, infraumbilical short vertical scar from previous umbilical location is strategically placed below the top bikini line

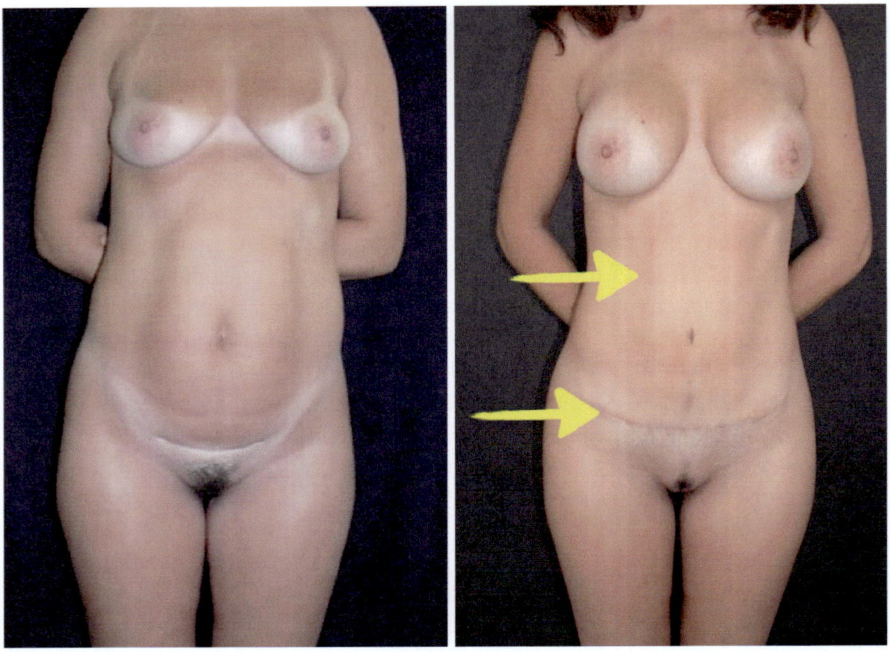

Fig. 7.2 (Slide 3 in PPT) – before and after combined procedure – abdominoplasty with repair of large rectus diastasis, liposuction of the back and flanks, and breast augmentation. *Arrows* from *top* to *bottom* outline, improvement of rectus lateral margin after diastasis repair; well-healed scar with excellent placement below the bikini line

7.4.1 Surgical Planning

Among our abdominoplasty patients, the most frequent request is for suction-assisted lipectomy (SAL) of adjacent areas including flanks, back, hips, and thighs.

In our practices, respectively, we routinely adjoin liposuction of the back and flank areas to our abdominoplasties. Starting in the prone position, the back and flank adiposities are addressed first prior to undertaking the anterior trunk. Circumferential reduction of excess adiposity produces a total torso transformation and improves the visual aesthetic from every angle. Liposuction of the back and flanks further assists in creating a defined waist where traditional abdominoplasty can blunt the waistline. Residual adiposity in the flanks and back can distract from an overall harmonious result from an abdominoplasty; when one area becomes smaller and tighter, it can call attention to other problem areas that were previously less noticeable.

Marking is done preoperatively while patient is standing. In all patients, we prefer abdominoplasty scar placed below the top bikini line. If umbilical scar cannot be removed completely, a short vertical scar is preferred instead of placing horizontal abdominoplasty scar in a higher level.

Things to Remember

- *We prefer abdominoplasty scar placed below the top bikini line. If umbilical scar cannot be removed completely, a short vertical scar is preferred instead of placing horizontal abdominoplasty scar in a higher level.*

7.4.2 Anesthesia

General anesthesia should always be used in body contouring procedures. Excellent control of the airway is critical since the patient is moved and turned many times during the procedure. Initially, patient is transferred from the stretcher to the surgical table by turning from supine to prone position to achieve the liposuction of the back area and later back to a supine position to continue with the abdominoplasty procedure. Compression boots (SCD's) are in place prior to induction, continued in the recovery room, and during the overnight stay. All patients are kept warmed with the use of a warm blanket and warm fluids. Hypothermia, a common problem in prolonged body contouring procedures with significant body exposure, can be completely avoided/prevented if appropriate preventative measures are taken at all times.

7.4.3 Patient Positioning

Once the patient is intubated and the endotracheal tube is secured, the patient is carefully placed in a prone position with padding under the arms, breast, and hips. The table is flexed and reversed Trendelenburg position is applied to avoid head down for prolonged periods and significant facial swelling. At this point, the tumescent solution is injected through one or two small incisions on the back. The superior midline incision is placed at the level of the brassiere, and the inferior midline incision at the top portion of the infra-gluteal fold. This process is followed by prepping and draping of the surgical area. After adequate time to allow the tumescent solution to work, the liposuction is completed in all of the pre-marked areas, using the power-assisted liposuction system. If fat injection is anticipated, fat collection is done during this part of the procedure (Fig. 7.3).

7.4.4 Patient Turning

Patient turning is a critical part of modern abdominoplasty surgery. It is done by a well-trained team in a safe and quick manner by protecting the airway, intravenous lines, and all patient extremities. We use a draw sheet and four team members to

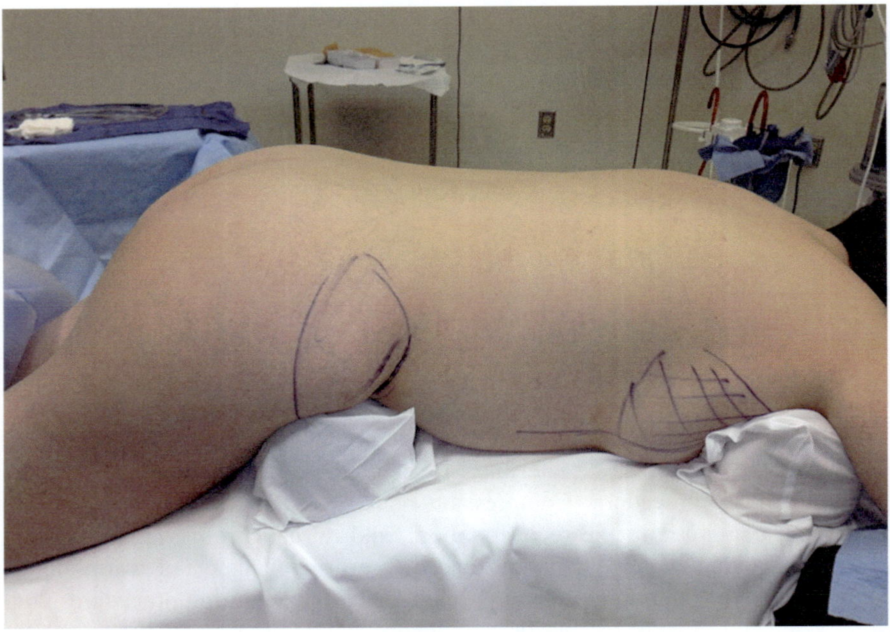

Fig. 7.3 (Slide 3 in PPT) – initial patient prone position ready for tumescent infiltration – surgical table flexed with padded hips, breasts, knees, and arms. Heating blanket is used *below* knees and *above* upper back immediately after patient is prepped

perform this part of the procedure. An effective and safe turning should be done in less than 15 s by protecting the patient, the airway, intravenous lines, and all other important accessories of the operation.

7.4.5 Surgical Technique

Once turning is completed, the abdominal markings are double-checked and only then injected with vasoconstriction solution. Patient is re-prepped and redraped. Team members scrub again and change gowns/gloves. Prior to making the first cut, symmetry is verified.

Anatomical details of importance in modern and safe abdominoplasty as emphasized by Saldanha [23, 24] include preservation of the Scarpa's fascia in the abdominal flap for increased blood supply to the dermis and skin. Also, by performing a selective tunnel undermining (instead of total undermining) over the rectus diastasis only preserving the lateral rectus muscle perforators, 80 % of the blood supply to the abdominal wall is protected. Thus, reducing complications when compared to traditional abdominoplasty and also combined bariatric surgery.

After liposuction is completed, abdominoplasty is carried out. Adding liposuction to abdominoplasty flap (lipoabdominoplasty) when necessary increases the pliability of the abdominoplasty flap and makes postoperative result better. Liposuction of the abdominal flap first also makes the elevation of the abdominal flap easier. Additionally, vasoconstrictor agents in liposuction solution spare the perforator vessels. The main concern with concurrent liposuction of the abdomen with abdominoplasty is ischemia and necrosis of the flap. The area most at risk for this complication is a triangular area beginning at the umbilicus and extending to the suprapubic region. When the perforator vessels are spared, we did not expect such a complication. And we did not observe such a complication in our cases, either.

During the dissection, a narrow undermining of the midline by preserving the lateral rectus muscle perforators is critical as described in the inverse abdominoplasty technique section. The supraumbilical tunnel is undermined all the way up to the xiphoid process, preserving the lateral neurovascular bundles that support the abdominal flap. Once the entire supraumbilical flap and the inferior flap are free, the pull-down approach is used to estimate where the inferior flap or the lower resection can be made end bloc and without much tension, and the rectus fascia plication is performed.

Things to Remember

- The *perforator vessels* are located consistently in a 2-cm radius located 4 cm from the midline and 6 cm from the subcostal margin [33].

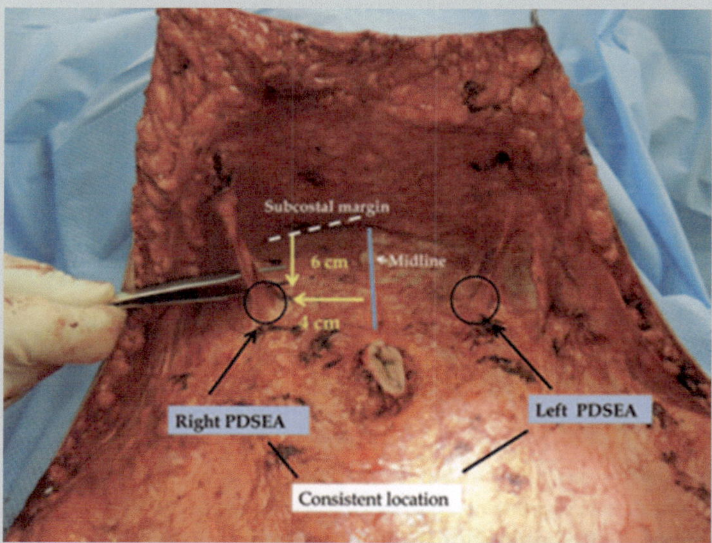

- *Lipoabdominoplasty* (described in 2001): Liposuction of the abdomen combined to rectus muscle plication through selective and safe undermining of the abdominal flap in the supraumbilical area by preserving the lateral rectus muscle perforators, thus increasing blood supply to the abdominal flap and its survival, decreasing the incidence of seroma and other complications of traditional abdominoplasty.

7.4.6 Pain Control, Drains

Before closing the lower abdominal wound, drains are placed, and injections of Exparel® (bupivacaine liposome injectable suspension) to the fascia are done. The drains are extended to the lower back and brought out through the suprapubic area. They drain the liposuctioned areas and lower abdomen, therefore decreasing the amount of swelling and bruising in the lower back. During the early postoperative period, we recommend the drains to be on low suction during recovery room and overnight admission.

If one elects to use Exparel®, the injections should follow manufacturers' recommendations and cover the rectus aponeurosis, external oblique aponeurosis (if the extended technique was used), and around the incision sites. Since senior author (RS) has been using Exparel® exclusively in all abdominoplasty cases and observed that patients have absolutely no abdominal pain and only some discomfort easily treatable with nonsteroidal anti-inflammatory drugs like ibuprofen, he has completely stopped the pain pumps usage.

Things to Remember

- Postoperative *pain control allows early ambulation*, thereby *decreases the theoretical potential of thrombophilia.*

7.4.7 Optimizing Outcomes

Promoting safe surgical practice and prevention of catastrophic events are the surest ways to optimize outcomes. Prior to the operating room, there should be a vigilant investigation of both personal and family history of thrombotic events. Our guidelines in clinical practice are as follows (Table 7.1):

Table 7.1 Our guidelines in clinical practice of combined abdominoplasty procedures (abdominoplasty + liposuction, abdominoplasty + aesthetic breast surgery, etc.)

Hematologic and/or appropriate specialist consultation for patient or family history of coagulopathy including miscarriages, early myocardial infarction, prior thromboembolic events
Cancelation of immediate preoperative trips via airplane or car
A baseline preoperative duplex scan with even a minor clinical suspicion
Oral contraceptives and hormones stopped at least a month prior to surgery
Sequential compression devices prior to induction of anesthesia, in recovery room, and during overnight stay
Adequate temperature management to avoid hypothermia
Low-molecular-weight heparins (Lovenox) starting at 8–10 h after completion of surgical procedure and to continue 3–5 days until fully ambulatory
Aggressive early ambulation by recovery room and overnight stay nurse personnel
Patient and family to be educated about the importance of ambulation in the immediate postoperative period so it continues at home after discharge from the surgical facility

An outstanding postoperative appearance does not guarantee that an outcome is satisfactory to the parties involved. A postoperative period that is free of major clinical complications and delayed healing can significantly enhance both patient and surgeon satisfaction.

7.4.8 Postoperative Care

All patients should be placed in a semi-compressive dressing after abdominoplasty and other ancillary procedures. Initial dressing with foam dressing such as Reston over liposuctioned areas and abdominal binders is appropriate. In our practice, patients are instructed to purchase compressive garments that encompass the abdomen and hips and wear the garments continuously for 6 weeks after surgery. Both medical grade and commercially available compressive garments are appropriate as long as they are worn with consistency. Surgical edema often persists for several months, and inconsistent use of garments can exacerbate the unflattering appearance.

Scar massage, lymphatic massage, and topical therapies such as silicone sheets are frequently used among our patients with the understanding that the therapeutic outcomes are highly variable. Frequent and regular postoperative visits are essential in impeding wound problems before they flare out of proportion.

Postsurgery weight control is regularly discussed with our patients so that the surgical results are maintained. This is especially crucial in the postoperative period when the patient may be more sedentary than usual, and activity restrictions prevent them from strenuous exercise.

Patients are kept in the surgery center overnight for safe postoperative management (pain control, fluid management, and deep vein thrombosis (DVT)/pulmonary embolism (PE) prevention) when abdominoplasty is combined with other body contouring procedures or patient's health conditions warrant closer observation and care. The compression girdle is recommended for the first 4–6 weeks. Patients are then allowed to resume regular exercises. Their weight is checked and documented in the chart during all office visits.

7.4.9 Complications

In the past, abdominoplasty has been implicated in higher incidence of complications when performed in a combined procedure. In the 2001, ASAPS Lipoplasty Survey performed between 1998 and 2000; data from 159 procedures was collected [32]. ASAPS members reported on 94,159 lipoplasty procedures. In all, 66 % of the procedures were suction-assisted lipectomy (SAL = lipoplasty = liposuction) alone, 20 % were lipoplasty without abdominoplasty but with one or more additional procedures, and 14 % of the SAL was combined with abdominoplasty. At result, they reported that the addition of abdominoplasty to suction-assisted lipectomy increased the likelihood of postoperative complications by a factor of 14. After this study was carried

Table 7.2 Combined surgeries of 175 lipoabdominoplasty patients

Combined surgeries of lipoabdominoplasty patients	175 patients
Only lipoabdominoplasty	34 (20 %)
Combined with SAL back/extremities	79 (46 %)
Combined with breast surgery	31 (17 %)
Combined with other surgeries	31 (17 %)

SAL suction assisted liposuction

out, lipoabdominoplasty concept has become popular which was based on the preservation of the perforator vessels, and thereby increasing the safety of the lipoabdominoplasty procedure and decreasing the complications accordingly [23, 24, 33]. Additionally, with implementation of safe clinical practices such as preoperative screening, effective pain control, early ambulation, and multiple methods of anticoagulation; complications including thromboembolic events observed after liposuction-abdominoplasty combination decreased at the last decades.

The development of deep vein thrombosis and pulmonary embolism poses a small but significant risk for surgical patients and may result in death or debilitating consequences. The risk of deep venous thrombosis (DVT) and pulmonary embolism (PE) in liposuction-abdominoplasty combination is likely multifactorial: prolonged operative time, increased pelvic vein compression due to rectus muscle diastasis repair which theoretically increases intra-abdominal pressure, and prolonged recovery period with relative immobility.

Muscle plication and abdominal binders that can compress the abdominal cavity may also interfere with respiratory mechanics. Changes in pulmonary compliance can occur after abdominal plication and may be predictive of respiratory complications. Rectus plication causing intraabdominal hypertension decreases venous return, results in venous stasis, and thus increased deep venous thrombosis risk occurs. A study conducted on 12 abdominoplasty patients confirmed the effect of rectus plication on increasing intraabdominal pressure but also implicated bed position, binder placement, and general anesthetic as risk factors [34]. Combination with the liposuction can worsen the vicious circle by increasing the immobility and edema. On the other hand, in other studies minimal changes in intraabdominal pressures and minimal to negligible changes in intrathoracic pressures were reported after abdominoplasty with muscle plication. It is important to note that pulmonary function assessed with pulmonary function tests and peak airway pressures may be insufficient measures of acute respiratory changes that could lead to postoperative pulmonary morbidity. Additionally, strength of plication is also important.

Over a 2-year period, 175 patients underwent lipoabdominoplasties in the senior author's (RS) practice. One hundred forty-one patients (80 %) underwent combination procedures (Table 7.2).

The complications of combined procedures were comparable to rates after lipoabdominoplasty alone and superior to rates associated with traditional abdominoplasty in the author's practice. Three patients required hospitalization after a combined procedure: two admissions were for postsurgical complications and one patient for inadvertent narcotic overdose while at home. There was a single incidence of pulmonary embolism that recovered well with intravenous heparin therapy

Table 7.3 Complications among 175 patients who underwent lipoabdominoplasty alone or in combination

Complications among 175 patients who underwent lipoabdominoplasty alone or in combination	
Seroma	5 (2.85 %)
Pulmonary embolism	1 (0.5 %)
Dehiscence	1 (0.5 %)
Narcotic overdose	1 (0.5 %)

and hospitalization. This particular patient received both mechanical and chemical prophylaxes. It was discovered afterwards that the patient had driven 10 h the day prior to surgery (Table 7.3).

The Authors' Comment By better preserving the nerves and vasculature to the anterior abdominal wall, modern abdominoplasty likely reduces much of the most common and aggravating complications of traditional abdominoplasty, including seromas and lower skin flap necrosis. When perforator vessels are spared, abdominoplasty can be safely combined with liposuction (liposuction of abdominal flap) with no increase in complication rates. This procedure can potentially be safely combined with other aesthetic procedures to produce a more dramatic transformation.

7.5 Abdominoplasty Combined with Aesthetic Breast Surgery

Among abdominoplasty patients, the second most frequent request is for aesthetic breast surgery. In this section, we address the issues surgeons facing in abdominoplasty – aesthetic breast surgery combination and the findings in the literature and our experience (RS and DO).

Among the weight loss and multiparous patients, the ptotic, involuted breasts can similarly detract from achieving a harmonious result. The huge popularity of the so-called mommy makeovers stems from the high incidence of simultaneous deformities of the breasts and the abdomen. Augmentation, mastopexy, and augmentation-mastopexy are the most common cosmetic breast operations combined with abdominoplasty to rejuvenate and restore felicitous dimensions to the breasts. When combined with lipoabdominoplasty and suction-assisted lipectomy of the lower torso, breast aesthetic surgery can facilitate a more complete transformation (Figs. 7.4 and 7.5) (Table 7.4).

7.5.1 Preoperative Planning and Surgical Technique

Matarasso and Smith [35] pointed out that "The operation performed on one site does not necessarily impact the other (i.e., tension on the abdominoplasty flap does not affect inframammary fold location)." We agree with this conclusion to some

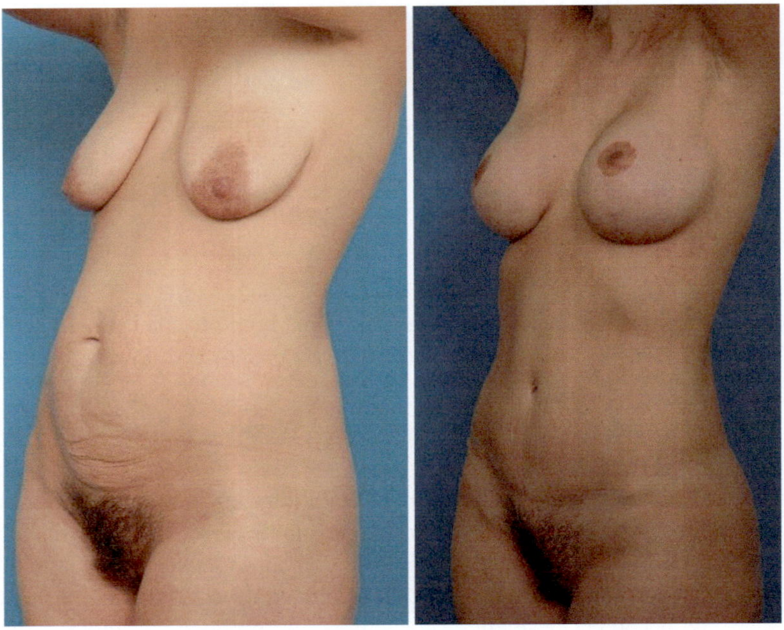

Fig. 7.4 (Slide 4–5 in PPT) – massive weight loss patient after combined procedures – modern safe abdominoplasty combined to breast augmentation, mastopexy, liposuction upper, lower back, and flanks

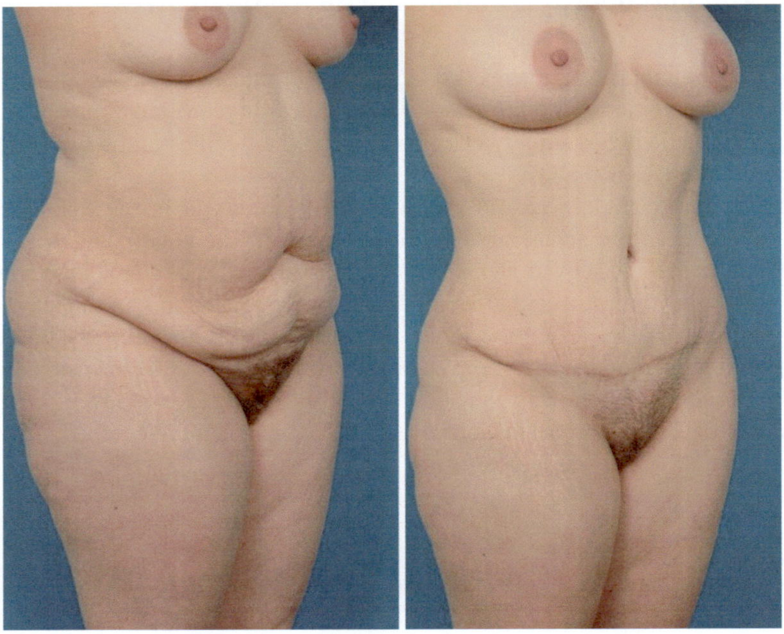

Fig. 7.5 (Slide 6–7 in PPT) – massive weight loss patient after combined procedures – breast augmentation, modern safe abdominoplasty, breast augmentation, liposuction of *upper*, *lower* back, and flanks

Table 7.4 Types of aesthetic breast surgery procedures in 268 patients [6] undergoing abdominoplasty and aesthetic breast surgery combination

Augmentation mammaplasty	69 patients (29 %)
Augmentation-mastopexy	75 patients (27 %)
Mastopexy alone	63 patients (23 %)
Reduction mammaplasty	46 patients (17 %)
Removal and replacement of breast implants	15 patients (6 %)

extent except in cases when one has to move down the inframammary fold, such as for tuberous breasts or some asymmetric breasts. In those cases, the inframammary fold is often difficult to position, so we believe that combined procedures can be avoided or planned accordingly. Similarly, in cases where a T-scar is used for mastopexy or reduction, a combined abdominoplasty can result in excessive traction on the sutures in the inframammary fold, which can increase the risk of wound dehiscence or hypertrophic scars, or postoperatively sliding of the scar below the fold can occur.

In such patients, extratension arisen from abdominoplasty should be taken into account during planning. Otherwise, patients can develop hypertrophic scars in the inframammary fold following combined surgery, attributed to excessive traction of the concomitant abdominoplasty. Our preference for breast reduction surgery and mastopexy is vertical scar technique. To prevent the passage of the vertical scar beyond the fold due to excessive tension arising from abdominoplasty, the vertical limbs of the drawing should join to each other 2–3 cm above the fold. If the case is a gigantomastia case, then vertical limbs of the drawing should be planned 4–5 cm above the fold to prevent the passage of the scar below the fold. If there is suspicion about the correct placement of the scar in T-scar reduction cases, starting with the abdominoplasty first then proceeding with the reduction mammaplasty can be more reasonable to place the horizontal limb of the T-scar in the inframammary fold precisely.

With a skilled team working in concert, we are generally able to complete the indicated breast procedure and abdominoplasty within approximately 4 h. My preference (DO) for breast reduction/mastopexy procedure is almost always vertical mammaplasty having superior or superomedial/superolateral pedicle [36]. Preoperatively, drawing is done while patient is standing. Information is given to the patient about the appearance of the scars. Extreme cases of abdominoplasty and reduction mammaplasty should be operated in different sessions (Figs. 7.6–7.8).

We (RS and DO) perform abdominoplasty as the last of multiple procedures because of the extreme beach chair flexion necessary to achieve maximal resection and have not found the abdominal closure to have an impact on the inframammary fold in non-massive weight loss patients. Measures to reduce the risk of systemic morbidity potentially increased by any combination surgery must be taken. Augmentation mammaplasty by reverse abdominoplasty (AMBRA) is best suited to those with predominantly *upper* abdominal laxity and adiposity who desire autologous tissue breast augmentation and/or mastopexy combined with reverse abdominoplasty [37].

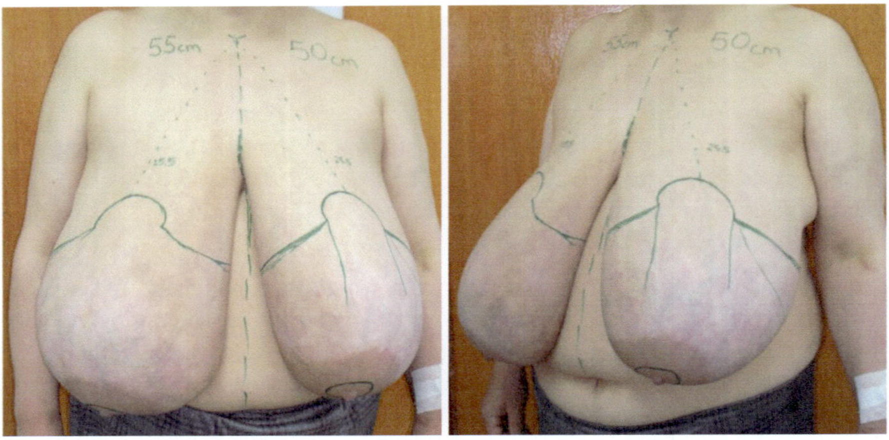

Fig. 7.6 Abdominal skin laxity, fat deposition and gigantomastia. Sternal nocth – nipple distance were 55 cm and 50 cm

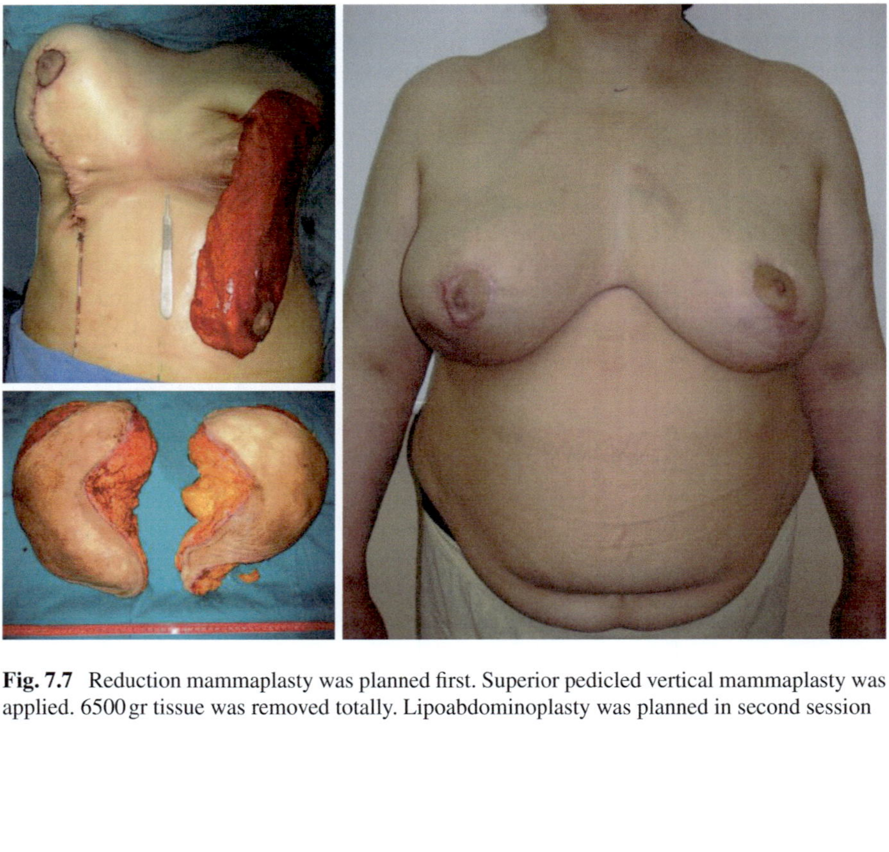

Fig. 7.7 Reduction mammaplasty was planned first. Superior pedicled vertical mammaplasty was applied. 6500 gr tissue was removed totally. Lipoabdominoplasty was planned in second session

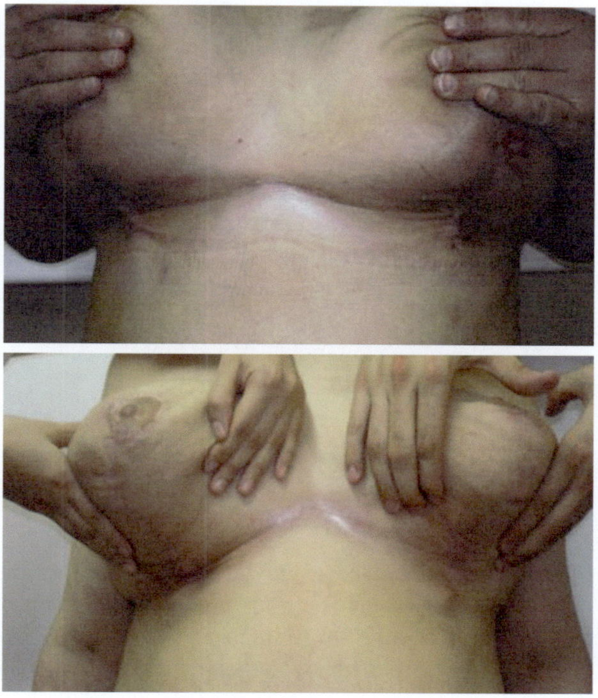

Fig. 7.8 Apperance of the vertical scar ending at the level of the fold

7.5.2 *Postoperative Care*

All patients should be placed in a semi-compressive dressing after abdominoplasty and aesthetic breast surgery procedures. In our practice, patients are instructed to purchase compressive bra and garments that encompass the breast at inframammary fold and abdomen and wear garments continuously for 6 weeks after surgery. Both medical grade and commercially available compressive garments are appropriate as long as they are worn with consistency. Surgical edema often persists for several weeks, and inconsistent use of garments can exacerbate the unflattering appearance.

Scar massage, lymphatic massage, and topical therapies such as silicone sheets are used among our patients, if necessary, with the understanding that the therapeutic outcomes are highly variable. Frequent wound checks and regular postoperative visits are essential in impeding wound problems before they flare out of proportion.

Patients are kept in the surgery center overnight for safe postoperative management (pain control, fluid management, and DVT/PE prevention) when abdominoplasty is combined with aesthetic breast surgery. Same precautions indicated in Table 7.1 are taken for abdominoplasty and aesthetic breast surgery combination as well.

Things to Remember

- Tension on the abdominoplasty flap does not necessarily affect *inframammary fold location* except in cases when one has to move down the inframammary fold, such as for tuberous breasts or some asymmetric breasts. In such cases, combined procedures can be avoided or planned accordingly.
- Combining abdominoplasty and breast procedures is *safe* in the majority of patients.

7.5.3 Complications

Stevens et al. conducted a study to review the safety and efficacy of a large number of combined abdominoplasty and breast surgery cases performed by a single plastic surgery practice in 2006 [38]. In that study, 151 patients undergoing combined abdominoplasty and breast surgery were compared to 264 patients undergoing abdominoplasty alone over a 15-year period (1989–2004) [38]. At result, no significant differences existed between the combined abdominoplasty and breast surgery groups and abdominoplasty alone group with regard to either minor or major complications.

At the same center, same group of plastic surgeons performed an update of this study [6]. During the 10-year period between 1997 and 2007, a total of 268 patients undergoing abdominoplasty and aesthetic breast surgery combination were included. The mean patient age was 42 years, the mean body mass index (BMI) was 25, and 8 % of patients were smokers. Pertinent intraoperative data showed that the average operative time was 165 min (range, 60–330 min), the number of patients who underwent concurrent lipoplasty was 207 (77 %), and the average lipoplasty aspirate volume for these patients was 1213 mL (range 200–4800 mL). All of the surgeries were performed by one of two plastic surgeons at a single outpatient surgery center. All patients had pneumatic compression devices placed before the induction of general anesthesia, which were maintained in the recovery room. All patients ambulated within 1 h of the conclusion of the operative procedure. The patients were then discharged to an aftercare facility with nursing supervision for at least one night. They ambulated at least once per hour that evening and several times per day in the ensuing days. The distribution of abdominoplasty procedures included lower (11 %), mini (2 %), full (86 %), reverse (1 %), and circumferential abdominoplasty (0 %) techniques. The distribution of cosmetic breast procedures included augmentation (28 %), mastopexy (22 %), augmentation-mastopexy (27 %), reduction (17 %), and the removal and replacement of implants (6 %). A retrospective review of 268 patients who underwent combined abdominoplasty and cosmetic

Table 7.5 Comparison of complication and revision rates of combined abdominoplasty and cosmetic breast procedures to the complication and revision rate of individually performed/staged procedures [6]

Procedure	Complication rate	Revision rate
Combined abdominoplasty and cosmetic breast surgery	34 %	13 %
Abdominoplasty performed separately	10–40 %	10–24 %
Cosmetic breast surgery performed separately	2–25 %	2–26 %
Augmentation mammaplasty	2–21 %	2–19 %
Augmentation-mastopexy	17–23 %	9–17 %
Reduction mammaplasty	15–25 %	11–26 %

breast surgery over a 10-year period found a 34 % overall complication rate including seroma and wound dehiscence but no thromboembolic events or death. Combining two procedures did not lead to an increase in complications when compared to individually staged procedures. The complication and revision rates of the combined surgery were similar to those reported for individually staged procedures (Table 7.5).

Another study searching the short-term complication rate of combining abdominoplasty and aesthetic breast surgery has been performed by Khavanin et al. [39]. In their study, all women undergoing abdominoplasty, panniculectomy, augmentation mammaplasty, and/or mastopexy in the TOPS database were identified. Demographics and outcomes for combined procedures were compared to individual procedures. Multiple logistic regressions provided adjusted odd ratios for the effect of a combined procedure on 30-day complications. Among combined procedures, a logistic regression model determined point values for pretreatment risk factors including diabetes (1 point), age over 53 (1), obesity (2), and 3+ ASA status (3), creating a 7-point pretreatment risk stratification tool. A total of 58,756 cases met inclusion criteria. At result, complication rates among combined procedures (9.40 %) were greater than those of aesthetic breast surgery (2.66 %; $p<.001$) but did not significantly differ from abdominal procedures (9.75 %; $p=.530$). Nearly 77 % of combined cases were classified as low risk (0 points total) with a 9.78 % complication rates. Medium-risk patients (1–3 points) had a 16.63 % complication rate and high-risk patients (4–7 points) 38.46 %. In conclusion, they thought that combining abdominal and breast procedures is safe in the majority of patients and does not increase 30-day complication rates. The risk stratification tool can continue to ensure favorable outcomes for patients who may desire a combined surgery.

7.6 Abdominoplasty Combined with Facial Aesthetic Surgery

Facial aesthetic surgery can be combined with modern abdominoplasty but with caution as to the length of the procedure. Patients often desire a combination procedure of the face (e.g., a rhytidectomy) that would necessitate significant operative time and would result in excessive operative time if combined with body contouring procedures. If the patient also desires breast surgery and/or extensive suction-assisted lipectomy, other aesthetic surgeries may be best performed on a separate date.

7.7 Abdominoplasty Combined with Intra-abdominal/ Pelvic Surgery

The concept of combining abdominoplasty with other procedures evolved when abdominal reshaping was performed in conjunction with anatomically proximate operations such as gynecologic or intra-abdominal surgery. Hester et al. first reported favorably on combining abdominoplasty with intra-abdominal, pelvic, or other aesthetic procedures, noting comparable complication rates and citing only obesity as a risk factor for unfavorable outcomes [17]. Other early reports were less encouraging. In 1986 at the University of Utah, Voss et al. demonstrated higher morbidity, longer operative times, increased blood loss, and increased hospital stays when abdominoplasty was combined with common gynecologic operations [40]. Voss and colleagues reported that 6.6 % of patients (5 out of 76 patients) undergoing combined abdominoplasty with a gynecologic procedure had a pulmonary embolism versus no patients undergoing a single procedure. 6.6 % was a very high incidence for pulmonary embolism. However, this clinical study was reviewed and repeated at the same institution by the senior author (RS) [41] 14 years later. There were no thromboembolic events after the same number of patients and similar cases. The early foreboding results are tempered by the realization that significant practice modifications have been enacted since these studies were performed. Beran [42] concluded that "comparison of DVT/PE [deep venous thrombosis/pulmonary embolism] rates in these combined procedures before and after the adoption of venous thromboembolism prophylaxis modalities is like comparing infection rates before and after the time of Fleming."

Local complications related to adjacent-combined procedures have also been addressed in the literature. In Ali's series, for example, combining abdominoplasty with cesarean section led to higher complication rates and inferior aesthetic results secondary to distorted local anatomy and compromised healing because of contamination [43].

Massenburg et al. [44] conducted a study to see the outcomes of the combined abdominoplasty (ABP)-hysterectomy (HYS) since this combination is being increasingly requested by patients. The authors reviewed the American College of Surgeons National Surgical Quality Improvement Program database and identified each ABP, HYS, and combined ABP-HYS performed between 2005 and 2012. The incidence of complications in each of the three procedures was calculated, and a multiplicative-risk model was used to calculate the probability of a complication for a patient undergoing distinct HYS and ABP on different dates. One-sample binomial hypothesis tests were performed to determine statistical significance. There were 1325 ABP cases, 12,173 HYS cases, and 143 ABP-HYS cases identified. At result, surgical complications occurred in 7.7% of patients undergoing an ABP-HYS while the calculated risk of a surgical complication was 12.5% ($p=0.0407$) for patients undergoing separate ABP and HYS procedures. The mean operative time was significantly lower for an ABP-HYS at 238 versus 270 min for separate ABP and HYS procedures ($p<0.0001$), and the mean time under anesthesia was significantly lower at 295 versus 364 min ($p<0.0001$). In conclusion, they thought that a combined ABP-HYS has a lower incidence of surgical complications than separate ABP and HYS procedures performed on different dates. These data should not encourage all patients to elect a combined ABP-HYS, if only undergoing a HYS, as the combined procedure is associated with increased risks when compared to either isolated individual procedure. However, in patients who are planning on undergoing both procedures on separate dates, a combined ABP-HYS is a safe option that will result in fewer surgical complications, less operative time, less time under anesthesia, and a trend toward fewer days in the hospital.

Fortunately, local problems that may arise during adjacent-combined procedures, such as wound contamination and excess tension, are fairly straightforward to conceptualize and therefore avoid. Coon et al. report that in the massive weight loss population, performing multiple procedures in the same operative setting increases the total number of complications for a given number of trips to the operating room, but the absolute number of complications is no greater than would be expected if all procedures had been performed individually [45].

Another study of 103 abdominoplasties combined with intra-abdominal surgeries including 67 tubal ligations, 34 total abdominal hysterectomies, and 2 cholecystectomies reported only two minor complications and no thromboembolic complications [46]. Early ambulation was applied and recommended at result [46].

Institutional changes implemented for combined gynecologic and plastic surgery procedures during the time interval included a more detailed preoperative screening, sequential compression devices in all cases, postoperative low-molecular-weight heparins in selective cases, early ambulation and discharge, and significant increase in outpatient surgery. The relatively recent addition of fascia injections of Exparel® in all abdominoplasty cases has allowed patients to ambulate earlier and with greater ease. Decreased narcotic intake was also observed, hastening patient mobility, and physical recovery.

Combining abdominoplasty with local procedures such as ventral hernia repair and umbilical herniorrhaphy is now often accepted.

Conclusion

Since no prospective studies or studies with high levels of evidence are available, the literature about the safety of the abdominoplasty-combined procedure is a little bit controversial. Nonetheless, the advantages of the combined procedures for the patient and surgical team are evident. However, in practice, this requires sufficient experience in abdominal procedures, liposuction, as well as the aesthetic breasts surgery techniques. Thus, it is best to reserve the combined procedure for patients with no comorbidities or history of thromboembolic disease and to avoid performing it in patients after massive weight loss who are at increased risk of complications.

Ultimately, a combined procedure should be attempted with a clean preoperative workup and by a surgical team who can complete multiple procedures in an efficient and timely fashion. Postoperative care should include instructions for early ambulation and adequate analgesia. Overnight stay is mandatory in our practice for all patients who undergo combined procedures in addition to lipoabdominoplasty or traditional abdominoplasty. Also, overnight stays are recommended for patients with any prior medical conditions or for significant blood loss, difficult pain control, or difficult recovery from anesthesia. The ASPS Patient Safety Committee guidelines detail guidelines for appropriate preoperative workup, patient selection, and perioperative management of risk factors. Consistent application of safe practices is paramount in maximizing positive outcomes and minimizing negative events.

Modern abdominoplasty is a powerful and safe body-sculpting tool. In combination with other body contouring procedures, it can lead to a comprehensive body transformation anatomically, physiologically, and psychologically. We attained significant series demonstrating that we can safely combine other procedures with abdominoplasty without multiplying the number of complications. With vigilant patient screening, preoperative planning, and aggressive postoperative management, we can safely and effectively perform modern abdominoplasty in combination with other procedures.

References

1. American Society for Aesthetic Plastic Surgery. 2015 National totals for cosmetic procedures. Available at: www.surgery.org. Accessed 27 June 2016.
2. Zhao Y, Encinosa W. Bariatric surgery utilization and out-comes in 1998 and 2004: statistical brief #23. In: Healthcare Cost and Utilization Project (HCUP) statistical briefs. Rockville: Agency for Health Care Policy and Research; 2007. p. 1–7.
3. American Society for Metabolic and Bariatric Surgery. American society for metabolic and bariatric surgery fact sheets: metabolic & bariatric surgery. Available at: http://asmbs.org/. Accessed 15 Dec 2014.
4. Neaman KC, Hansen JE. Analysis of complications from abdominoplasty: a review of 206 cases at a university hospital. Ann Plast Surg. 2007;58:292–8.
5. Stevens WG, Cohen R, Vath SD, Stoker DA, Hirsch EM. Does lipoplasty really add morbidity to abdominoplasty? Revisiting the controversy with a series of 406 cases. Aesthet Surg J. 2005;25:353–8.
6. Stevens WG, Repta R, Pacella SJ, et al. Safe and consistent outcomes of successfully combining breast surgery and abdominoplasty: an update. Aesthet Surg J. 2009;29:129–34.
7. Winocour J, Gupta V, Ramirez JR, Shack RB, Grotting JC, Higdon KK. Abdominoplasty: risk factors, complication rates, and safety of combined procedures. Plast Reconstr Surg. 2015;136:597e–606e.
8. Grazer FM. Abdominoplasty. Plast Reconstr Surg. 1973;51:617–23.
9. Hensel JM, Lehman Jr JA, Tantri MP, Parker MG, Wagner DS, Topham NS. An outcomes analysis and satisfaction survey of 199 consecutive abdominoplasties. Ann Plast Surg. 2001;46:357–63.

10. Stewart KJ, Stewart DA, Coghlan B, Harrison DH, Jones BM, Waterhouse N. Complications of 278 consecutive abdominoplasties. J Plast Reconstr Aesthet Surg. 2006;59:1152–5.
11. Byrd HS, Barton FE, Orenstein HH, et al. Safety and efficacy in an accredited outpatient plastic surgery facility: a review of 5316 consecutive cases. Plast Reconstr Surg. 2003;112:636–41; discussion 642.
12. Matarasso A. Discussion: is it safe to combine abdominoplasty with elective breast surgery? a review of 151 consecutive cases. Plast Reconstr Surg. 2006;118:213–4.
13. Saad AN, Parina R, Chang D, Gosman AA. Risk of adverse outcomes when plastic surgery procedures are combined. Plast Reconstr Surg. 2014;13:1415–22.
14. Swanson E. Does combining abdominoplasty and liposuction really increase the risk of venous thromboembolism? Plast Reconstr Surg. 2015;136:402e–4e.
15. Swanson E. Prospective outcome study of 360 patients treated with liposuction, lipoabdominoplasty, and abdominoplasty. Plast Reconstr Surg. 2012;129:965–78; discussion 979–80.
16. Swanson E. Prospective clinical study of 551 cases of liposuction and abdominoplasty performed individually and in combination. Plast Reconstr Surg Glob Open. 2013;1:e32.
17. Hester TR, Baird W, Bostwick 3rd J, Nahai F, Cukic J. Abdominoplasty combined with other major surgical procedures: safe or sorry? Plast Reconstr Surg. 1989;83:997–1004.
18. Swanson E. Prospective photographic measurement study of 196 cases of breast augmentation, mastopexy, augmentation/mastopexy, and breast reduction. Plast Reconstr Surg. 2013;131:802e–19e.
19. Soltani AM, Keyes GR, Singer R, Reed L, Fodor PB. Outpatient surgery and sequelae: an analysis of the AAAASF Internet-based quality assurance and peer review database. Clin Plast Surg. 2013;40:465–73.
20. Illouz YG. A new safe and aesthetic approach to suction abdominoplasty. Aesthetic Plast Surg. 1992;16:237–45.
21. Matarasso A. Abdominolipoplasty: a system of classification and treatment for combined abdominoplasty and suction-assisted lipectomy. Aesthetic Plast Surg. 1991;15:111–21.
22. Matarasso A. Liposuction as an adjunct to a full abdominoplasty. Plast Reconstr Surg. 1995;95:829–36.
23. Saldanha OR, Pinto EB, Matos Jr WN, Lucon RL, Magalhães F, Bello EM. Lipoabdominoplasty without undermining. Aesthet Surg J. 2001;21:518–26.
24. Saldanha OR, Federico R, Daher PF, Malheiros AA, Carneiro PR, Azevedo SF, Saldanha Filho OR, Saldanha CB. Lipoabdominoplasty. Plast Reconstr Surg. 2009;124:934–42.
25. Matarasso A. Evaluation & techniques in abdominal contour surgery. In: Newman HM, editor. Plastic surgery educational foundation instructional course. Mosby: St. Louis; 1993. p. 1–17.
26. Matarasso A. Liposuction as an adjunct to a full abdominoplasty revisited. Plast Reconstr Surg. 2000;106:1197–202; discussion 1203.
27. Ousterhout DK. Combined suction-assisted lipectomy, surgical lipectomy, and surgical abdominoplasty. Ann Plast Surg. 1990;24:126–32; discussion 132.
28. Dillerud E. Abdominoplasty combined with suction lipoplasty: a study of complications, revisions, and risk factors in 487 cases. Ann Plast Surg. 1990;25:333–8; discussion 339.
29. Arthurs ZM, Cuadrado D, Sohn V, et al. Post-bariatric panniculectomy: pre-panniculectomy body mass index impacts the complication profile. Am J Surg. 2007;193:567–70; discussion 570.
30. Bertheuil N, Thienot S, Huguier V, Ménard C, Watier E. Medial thighplasty after massive weight loss: are there any risk factors for postoperative complications? Aesthetic Plast Surg. 2014;38:63–8.
31. Masoomi H, Paydar KZ, Wirth GA, Aly A, Kobayashi MR, Evans GR. Predictive risk factors of venous thromboembolism in autologous breast reconstruction surgery. Ann Plast Surg. 2014;72:30–3.
32. Hughes 3rd CE. Reduction of lipoplasty risks and mortality: an ASAPS survey. Aesthet Surg J. 2001;21:120–7.
33. Smith LF, Smith Jr LF. Safely combining abdominoplasty with aggressive abdominal liposuction based on perforator vessels: technique and a review of 300 consecutive cases. Plast Reconstr Surg. 2015;135:1357–66.

34. Huang GJ, Bajaj AK, Gupta S, Petersen F, Miles DA. Increased intraabdominal pressure in abdominoplasty: delineation of risk factors. Plast Reconstr Surg. 2007;119:1319–25.
35. Matarasso A, Smith DM. Combined breast surgery and abdominoplasty: strategies for success. Plast Reconstr Surg. 2015;135:849e–60e.
36. Ozçelik D, Unveren T, Toplu G, Bilgen F, Iskender A, Senyuva C. Vertical mammaplasty for gigantomastia. Aesthetic Plast Surg. 2009;33:246–9.
37. Zienowicz RJ, Karacaoglu E. Augmentation mammaplasty by reverse abdominoplasty (AMBRA). Plast Reconstr Surg. 2009;124:1662–72.
38. Stevens WG, Cohen R, Vath SD, Steven D, Stoker DA, Hirsch EM. Is it safe to combine abdominoplasty with elective breast surgery? A review of 151 consecutive cases. Plast Reconstr Surg. 2006;118:207–12.
39. Khavanin N, Jordan SW, Vieira BL, Hume KM, Mlodinow AS, Simmons CJ, Murphy Jr RX, Gutowski KA, Kim JY. Combining abdominal and cosmetic breast surgery does not increase short-term complication rates: a comparison of each individual procedure and pretreatment risk stratification tool. Aesthet Surg J. 2015;35:999–1006.
40. Voss SC, Sharp HC, Scott JR. Abdominoplasty combined with gynecological surgical procedures. Obstet Gynecol. 1986;67:181–5.
41. Saltz R. Two position comprehensive approach to abdominoplasty. Clin Plast Surg. 2014;41:681–704. Review.
42. Beran SJ. Combination procedures: balancing risk and reward. Aesthet Surg J. 2006;26:443.
43. Ali A, Essam A. Abdominoplasty combined with cesarean delivery: evaluation of the practice. Aesthetic Plast Surg. 2011;35:80–6.
44. Massenburg BB, Sanati-Mehrizy P, Ingargiola MJ, Rosa JH, Taub PJ. Outcomes and safety of the combined abdominoplasty-hysterectomy: a preliminary study. Aesthetic Plast Surg. 2015;39:667–73.
45. Coon D, Michaels JV, Gusenoff JA, Purnell C, Friedman T, Rubin JP. Multiple procedures and staging in the massive weight loss population. Plast Reconstr Surg. 2010;125:691–8.
46. Gemperli R, Neves RI, Tuma Jr P, Bonamichi GT, Ferreira MC, Manders EK. Abdominoplasty combined with other intraabdominal procedures. Ann Plast Surg. 1992;29:18–22.

Chapter 8
Umbilicus Management – History and New Trends: Creating a Neo-umbilicus

Kai Uwe Schlaudraff

The '*rotated Y*' *neo-umbilicoplasty* is a versatile and constraint-free design for an aesthetic belly button during Tiryaki's 'inverse' abdominoplasty or classic 'inferior' abdominoplasty.

After the *resection of the existing umbilical stalk* and full advancement of the abdominal flap, a *triple dermal flap in Y-shape* is designed at the desired location. *Defatting* of the umbilical area is carried beyond the bases of the dermal flaps and creates the *umbilical concavity. Periumbilical quilting sutures* provide efficient 'high tension' anchoring of the abdominal flap and *desepidermization of the tip of the superior flap* allows for efficient 'turnover' fixation of the neo-umbilicus. The *size* and *shape* of the neo-umbilicus can be *modified* by the *length of the branches of the Y-design*, the *amount of upward rotation* and the degree of *lower central tightening*.

Tie-over dressings are not necessary, healing is quick and the *scar* is *discreetly hidden* in the centre of the belly button.

8.1 The Umbilicus: Key Feature of the Aesthetic Abdomen

The umbilicus is the only physiologic scar of the human body that normally remains after birth and is considered a key component of the abdomen – both aesthetically and symbolically. This remainder scar of the umbilical cord serves as a central visual reference point and defines the supra-umbilical median sulcus. It also relates to the tendinous intersections of the straight abdominal muscles and transitions into the infraumbilical curvature of the abdomen.

K.U. Schlaudraff
Concept-Clinic, Plastic, Reconstructive and Aesthetic Surgery, Geneva, Switzerland
e-mail: schlaudraff@concept-clinic.ch

K.T. Tiryaki (ed.), *Inverse Abdominoplasty*, DOI 10.1007/978-3-319-39310-0_8

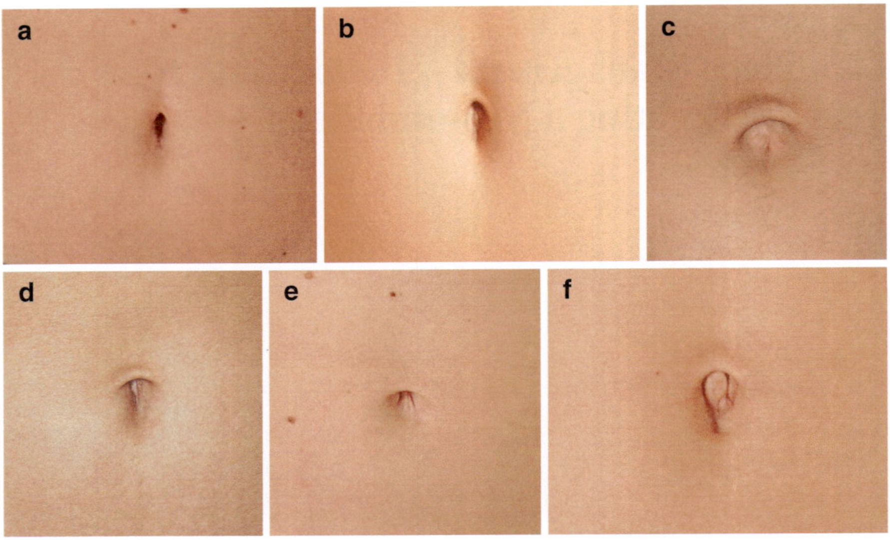

Fig. 8.1 (**a**) 'Vertical lozenge, (**b**) 'oval vertical with superior hooding', (**c**) 'round with superior hooding', (**d**) 'T-shaped with superior hooding', (**e**) 'oval horizontal with superior hooding', (**f**) 'protruded navel/outie with or without superior hooding'

Due to its central position, deformities of the navel, malpositions or its complete absence are instantly recognized as unnatural and create significant emotional distress for the patients [1–3].

As described by Kelly in 1899 [4], abdominoplasties had been successfully performed for more than a century, but at that time, the surgeons simply discarded the umbilicus – thus creating unattractive results. Alternatively, they buried the umbilicus under the abdominal flap – causing chronic omphalitis due to material accumulation [5, 6].

In the 1950s, Andrews presented his 'onfaloplastia' [7] and Vernon published the 'umbilical transplantation upward' – thus initiating the modern abdominoplasty technique based on transposition and reimplantation of the umbilicus into the lowered abdominal flap [3].

8.2 Aesthetic Considerations: Shape, Size and Positioning

The 'ideal' umbilicus measures 1.5–2 cm in diameter and is anatomically defined as abdominal midline structure of the linea alba. Craig et al. developed a classification of the umbilicus according to the shape, orientation and presence of 'hooding' [8] (Fig. 8.1).

The surrounding abdominal adipo-dermal flap transitions into the umbilicus through a characteristic periumbilical concavity that is deepest at the 12 o'clock position and less pronounced in the lateral and inferior periumbilical aspects. This 'horseshoe' shaped distribution of the fatty tissue is believed by Rozen and Redett to be an essential aesthetic feature ensuring overall abdominal beauty [9].

However, the presence of an exceedingly small size, an outward skin protrusion or an umbilical hernia is unanimously considered unattractive [10, 11].

The most appealing umbilicus – despite ethnic and cultural variations – is supposed to be small in size, with a vertical or T-shape and superiorly hooded. In a recent study on international multiethnic bikini models, the most appreciated navel shape was confirmed to be the vertical oval with superior hooding (82 %) and the least appreciated were the horizontal oval (29 %) and the protruding shape (47 %) [12].

Usually, surgeons position the umbilicus by retrieving the original projection of the umbilicus stalk and reimplanting the umbilicus into the lowered abdominal flap with the patient in neutral position. This approximates in patients with normal height (145–178 cm) to an average distance of 15 cm from the pubic symphysis [13] or to Fibonacci's 'golden ratio' of 1.618 of the distance xiphoid-umbilicus to umbilicus-abdominal crease [12].

In the author's opinion, proper positioning needs to take into account: (1) the height of the patient, (2) the initial natural position of the umbilicus, (3) the amount of mobilization and lowering of the abdominal flap, (4) the management of residual tension of the lowered flap using quilting sutures and (5) the fixation of the periumbilical abdominal flap on the fascia. All these factors influence the stability of the abdominal reshaping and determine the final outcome and shape of the umbilicus.

8.3 Transposition of the Original Umbilicus Versus A

8.3.1 Neo-umbilicus: Pros and Cons

'*The umbilicus is simply a scar and it would appear to be elementary especially for a plastic surgeon to replace one scar by another despite the sacred and almost mystical significance of the first*' (Yves-Gérard Illouz) [14].

Ever since Vernon's first transpositions of the umbilicus [3], a wide variety of designs for both umbilicus dissection and insets have been developed.

Baroudi initially described insetting the ovally excised umbilicus through a 2.5 cm horizontal incision in the abdominal flap that was conically defatted around the new umbilicus site [15]. He then revised his technique – adding two buried 3.0 non-absorbable sutures from the umbilical stalk to the fascia for pedicle shortening and a vertical skin incision for a more aesthetically pleasing umbilicus inset [10].

In the following, many more techniques were described – highlighting the ongoing quest for an optimal aesthetic solution but also the lack of a consensus between surgeons:

Avelar published a star-shaped incision [16], Juri et al. described the V-shaped incision [17] and Massiha combined a circular umbilical incision with a trilateral incision in the abdominal flap [18]. There are also reports of inverted U-shaped flap insets [19], inverted-V chevron umbilicoplasty [20] or Y-shaped deepithelialized skin flaps [21].

The fixation of the umbilical stalk onto the fascia is believed to shorten it sufficiently. This manoeuvre also improves the transition between the navel and the surrounding abdominal flap and enhances the periumbilical concavities. However, in case of elongated umbilical stalks, a shortening is mandatory in order to avoid a 'pleating' of excess skin and a 'pseudo'-herniation resulting in an unpleasant appearance. Akbas reported his solution to the problem through a vertical elliptical skin excision, embedding of the elongated stalk in the rectus abdominis muscles and suturing the abdominal skin at the 3, 6, 9 and 12 o'clock position to the fascia followed by a supra-umbilical liposuction – hereby improving the midline definition [6].

Visconti added four cardinal 3.0 absorbable stitches to his omphaloplasty, and performed an inferior-based triangular incision on the abdominal skin combined with a navel excision in a triangular shape with the apex pointing downward [12].

The author believes that despite thorough technical execution, many of the 'umbilical transposition' techniques are bound to the following challenges:

- Circular or elliptic excisions of the umbilicus often lead to scar retraction with subsequent stenosis and reduction of the size of the navel – which is commonly perceived as unaesthetic.
- Placing the scars for the umbilical inset on the periphery of the navel reveals them to the observer – especially in case of a hypertrophic scar reaction.
- Maintaining the umbilical stalk and its vascularization sometimes proves to be difficult – especially when a long umbilical stalk, large hernias or a wide diastasis are encountered.
- The efficiency of hernia repair or diastasis correction may be jeopardized because the surgeon needs to control the compression of the umbilical stalk vessels and may not perform fully sufficient continuous closure.
- Techniques burying a long umbilical stalk within the plication of the rectus abdominis muscle or fixating it to the fascia risks a delayed protrusion of the umbilical stalk with a 'cauliflower-like' appearance.

For the above reasons, the author has modified his personal technique for a routine excision of the umbilicus at its abdominal wall root followed by a full 'rotated Y' neo-umbilicoplasty.

8.4 Neo-umbilicoplasty Through a 'Rotated Y' Design

Based on the initial 4-flap design described by Cló et al. [11] and Lee et al. [22], the author designed and now routinely uses a 'rotated Y' design.

1. *Dissection*: after the routine dissection of the abdominal flap, the umbilical pedicle is excised and diastasis correction is performed with inverted X-stitches of PDS 0 absorbable monofilament sutures. Similar to the Tiryaki's triple spring

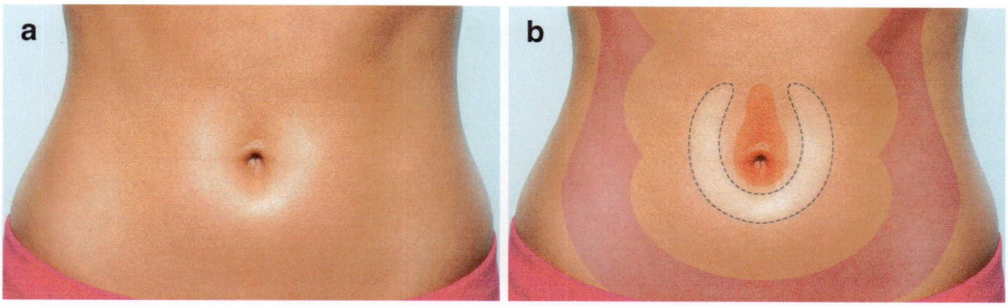

Fig. 8.2 (**a**) The 'perfect abdomen' with a 'horseshoe'-shaped distribution of periumbilical fat highlighted through the reflected flashlight. (**b**) The 'perfect abdomen' with its 'horseshoe'-shaped positive volume, peripheral shadows (*pink*) and umbilical concavity (*red*)

sutures, this technique provides both horizontal tightening and vertical shortening of the abdominal fascia.

2. *Placement*: the patient is placed in neutral – not 30° flexed – position, the abdominal flap is fully advanced and central closure is temporarily performed with staples. *This temporarily puts the abdominal flap under pronounced tension, mimics the 'high tension suture' effect and allows for umbilical placement approximately 1–1.5 cm higher on the abdominal flap*. Then, the correct placement of the neo-umbilicus in the midline is defined and the initial position of the umbilical stalk is retrieved on the abdominal wall and transcribed onto the advanced flap. *The skin incision is performed according to a 'rotated Y' design with the upper branches measuring 1.0 cm and the lower branch measuring 0.5 cm.*
3. *Defatting*: the triangular skin flaps are defatted fully until the dermal level and slightly beyond their respective bases – creating the deep central depression of the umbilicus. Care is taken to ensure a smooth transition from the 'horseshoe' shaped fatty volume of the surrounding abdominal flap to the deep centre of the umbilicus (Fig. 8.2). Furthermore, it is important to defat the superior skin flap 2–3 cm until the supra-umbilical zone in order to transition smoothly to the epigastric area that was treated through liposuction.
4. *Fixation*: four 2.0 absorbable monofilament sutures are placed from the tip of each skin flap to the aponeurosis at the 'natural' umbilicus position. The upper V-shaped flap is desepidermized in its tip and advanced slightly more superiorly – thus ensuring cutaneous hood creation. Both lateral flaps are advanced with an upward rotation and fixated through another stitch from the aponeurosis to the tip of each flap. This manoeuvre allows for correction of the diameter of the neo-umbilicus – more rotation tightens the diameter and results in a more oval shape. Skin closure is performed through simple sutures with Prolene 5.0.
5. *Dressing*: due to the strong fixation of the neo-umbilicus on the abdominal wall, a simple dressing with Jelonet and cotton gauzes is sufficient (Fig. 8.3, 8.4, 8.5, and 8.6).

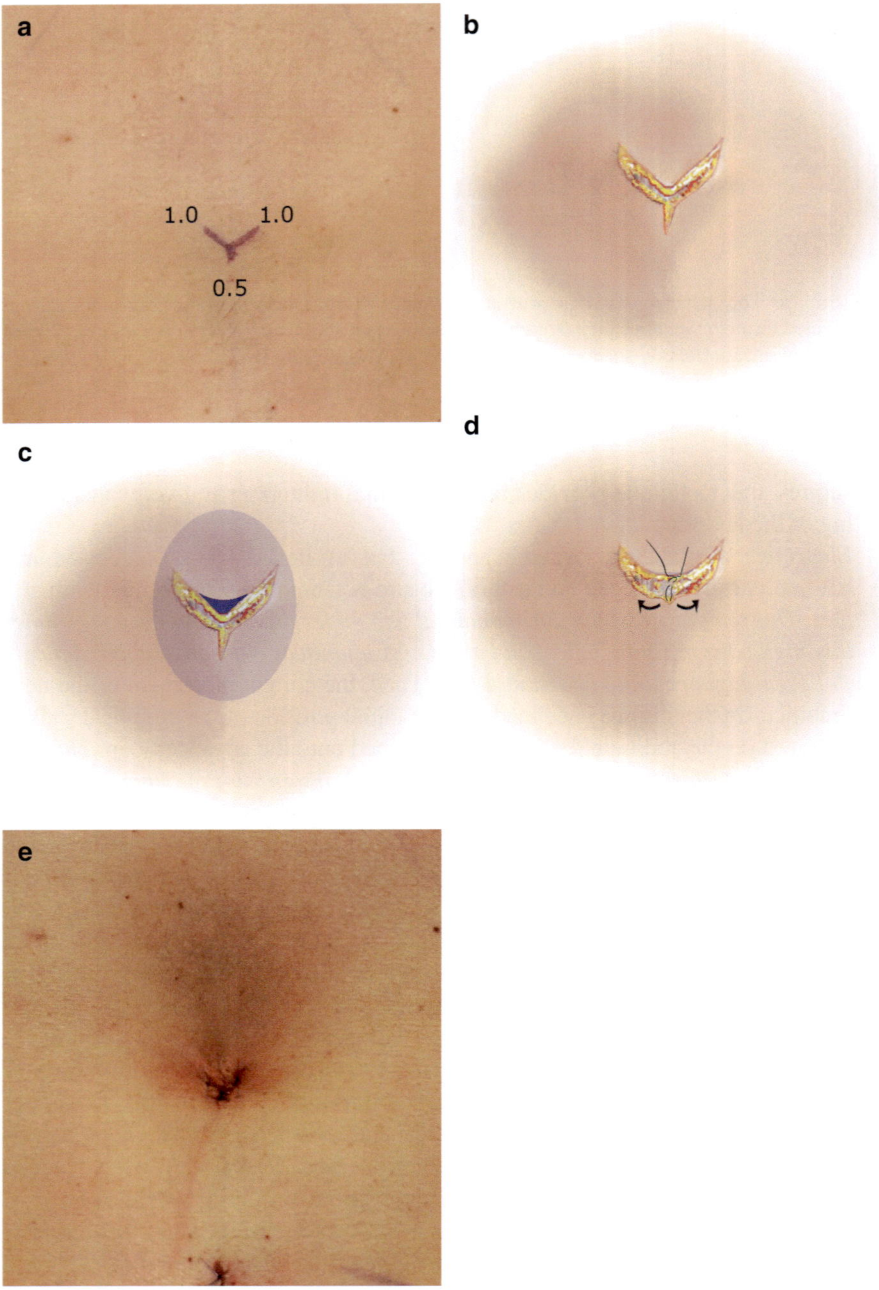

Fig. 8.3 (**a**) Flap design for neo-umbilicoplasty. (**b**) The skin is incised and three triangular flaps are raised. (**c**) Defatting is done in an oval shape (*light blue*) and desepidermization of the tip of the superior flap is performed (*dark blue*). (**d**) The superior flap is folded inside, internally fixated on the aponeurosis with a 2.0 absorbable monofilament and sutured to the base of the Y-shape. This creates an upward move and a rotation of each lower flap laterally (*arrows*). (**e**) Final result after fixation and skin closure

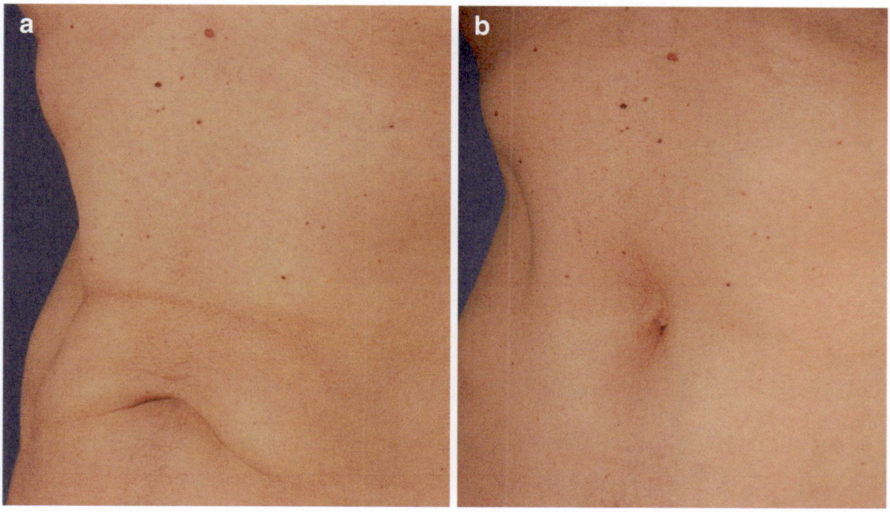

Fig. 8.4 (**a**) Patient 1: massive weight loss patient – preoperative oblique view. (**b**) Patient 1: postoperative oblique view at 1 month

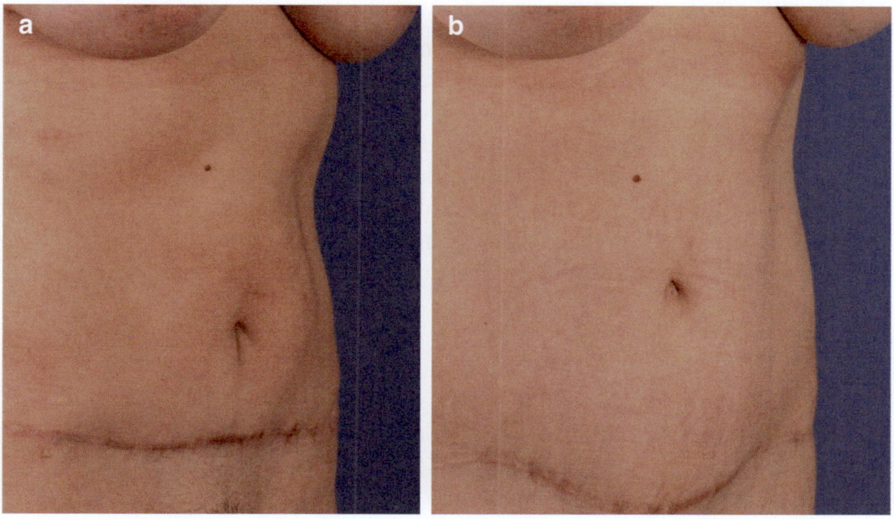

Fig. 8.5 (**a**) Patient 2: revision abdominoplasty – preoperative oblique view. (**b**) Patient 2: postoperative oblique view at 9 months

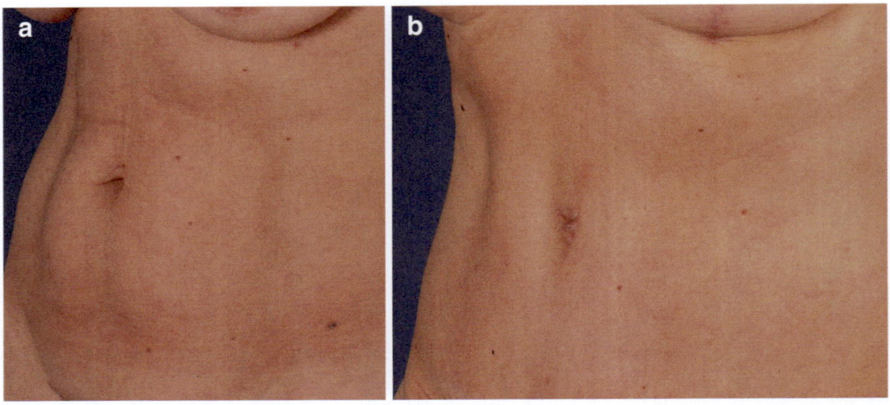

Fig. 8.6 (**a**) Patient 3: 'mommy makeover' – preoperative oblique view. (**b**) Patient 3: postoperative oblique view at 6 months

8.5 Advantages of the 'Rotated Y' Neo-umbilicoplasty

For the surgeon:

- Easy abdominal and umbilical dissection
- Efficient management of hernias or muscle diastasis
- Simple repositioning of the neo-umbilicus without constraints
- Secure fixation through a large zone of dermo-fascial adherence
- Maintained vascularization of the skin flaps avoiding wound healing problems
- No need for tie-over dressings thus avoiding skin maceration
- Efficient periumbilical volume management
- Secure creation of the central depression of the umbilicus creating an harmonious abdomen

For the patient:

- Hidden scar placement avoiding telltale signs of surgery
- Recreation of a slim waistline through efficient retightening of the abdominal wall muscles
- Aesthetically pleasing and stable result

8.6 Conclusion

The 'rotated Y' neo-umbilicoplasty offers technical ease of surgical dissection, facilitates hernia repair and correction of abdominal muscle diastasis and allows for efficient 'high tension' anchoring of the neo-umbilicus and the surrounding abdominal flaps through umbilical key-stitches and periumbilical quilting sutures.

The location of the neo-umbilicus can be chosen without constraints and the design can be modified easily to achieve the desired length and width of belly button.

In the author's opinion, it is the perfect complement to Tiryaki's 'inverse abdominoplasty' technique combining safety, surgical efficacy with a superior aesthetic outcome.

Points to Remember

Flaws of transposed belly buttons:

- External periumbilical scars are most often aesthetically unsatisfactory
- Oval or circular insets usually retract to a small-sized umbilicus
- Delayed protrusion of umbilical stalks often occurs even with deep fixation – this results in an unpleasant, 'outie' look
- The preserved umbilical stalk often interferes with hernia or diastasis correction or is put at risk for ischemia and wound healing problems in case of tight repair

Pearls of the 'rotated Y' neo-umbilicoplasty:

- Hidden scar placement is ensured
- Turnover fixation of the desepidermized tip of the cranial V-flap combined with periumbilical quilting sutures provides secure anchoring of both umbilicus and abdominal flap
- Tie-over dressings are not needed
- The vertical size of the neo-umbilicus can be modified through lengthening the upper and lower, 'branches' or applying a steeper angle of the Y-design

References

1. Hakme F. Abdominoplasty: peri- and supra-umbilical lipectomy. Aesthetic Plast Surg. 1983;7:213–20.
2. Regnault P. The history of abdominal dermolipectomy. Aesthetic Plast Surg. 1978;2:113–23.
3. Vernon S. Umbilical transplantation upward and abdominal contouring in lipectomy. Am J Surg. 1957;96:490–9.
4. Kelly HA. Report of gynecological cases. Johns Hopkins Med J. 1899;10:197.
5. Baack BR, Anson G, Nachbar JM, White DJ. Umbilicoplasty: the construction of a new umbilicus and correction of umbilical stenosis without external scars. Plast Reconstr Surg. 1996;97:227–31.
6. Akbas H, Guneren E, Eroglu L, Uysal OA. Natural-looking umbilicus as an important part of abdominoplasty. Aesthetic Plast Surg. 2003;27:139–42.
7. Andrews JM. Nova tecnica de lipectomia abdominal e onfaloplastia. Memoria do VIII Cong Lat Am Cir Plast, Cuba. 1956.
8. Craig SB, Faller MS, Puckett CL. In search of the ideal female umbilicus. Plast Reconstr Surg. 2000;105:389.

9. Rozen SM, Redett R. The two-dermal-flap umbilical transposition: a natural and aesthetic umbilicus after abdominoplasty. Plast Reconstr Surg. 2007;119:2255–62.
10. Baroudi R. Umbilicoplasty. Clin Plast Surg. 1975;2:431–48.
11. Cló TCT, Nogueira DSC. A New umbilical reconstruction technique used for 306 consecutive abdominoplasties. Aesthetic Plast Surg. 2012;36(5):1009–14.
12. Visconti G, Visconti E, Bonomo L, Salgarello M. Concepts in navel aesthetic: a comprehensive surface anatomy analysis. Aesthetic Plast Surg. 2014;39(1):43–50.
13. Rodriguez-Feliz JR, Makhijani S, Przybyla A, Hill D, Chao J. Intraoperative assessment of the umbilicopubic distance: a reliable anatomic Landmark for transposition of the umbilicus. Aesthetic Plast Surg. 2011;36(1):8–17.
14. Illouz YG. A new safe and aesthetic approach to suction abdominoplasty. Aesthetic Plast Surg. 1992;16:237–45.
15. Baroudi R, Keppke EM, Netto FT. Abdominoplasty. Plast Reconstr Surg. 1974;54:161–8.
16. Avelar JM. Abdominoplasty: technical refinement and analysis of 130 cases in 8 years' follow-up. Aesthic Plastic Surg. 1983;7:205–12.
17. Juri J, Juri C, Raiden G. Reconstruction of the umbilicus in abdominoplasty. Plast Reconstr Surg. 1979;63:580–2.
18. Massiha H, Montegut W, Phillips R. A method of reconstructing a natural-looking umbilicus in abdominoplasty. Ann Plast Surg. 1997;38:228–31.
19. Malic CC, Spyrou GE, Hough M, Fourie L. Patient satisfaction with two different methods of umbilicoplasty. Plast Reconstr Surg. 2007;119:357–61.
20. Lesavoy MA, Fan K, Guenther DA, Herrera F, Little JW. The inverted-V chevron umbilicoplasty for breast reconstruction and abdominoplasty. Aesthet Surg J. 2012;32(1):110–6.
21. Castillo PF, Sepulveda CA, Prado AC, Troncoso AL, Villaman JJ. Umbilical reinsertion in abdominoplasty: technique using deepithelialized skin flaps. Aesthetic Plast Surg. 2007;31:519–20.
22. Lee YT, Kwon C, Rhee SC, Cho SH, Eo SR. Four flaps technique for neoumbilicoplasty. Arch Plast Surg. 2015;42(3):351.

Chapter 9
Abdominal Wall Hernias and Their Repair with Inverse Abdominoplasty

Ozay Ozkaya Mutlu, Ozlem Colak, and Murat Atay

9.1 Introduction

The abdominal wall is made up of muscles that mirror of each other from right to left. These include rectus abdominis, external oblique, internal oblique and the transversalis. Hernia is derived from a Latin word means “rupture” [1]. The definition of a hernia of the abdominal wall is an abnormal protrusion of the abdominal contents through an acquired or congenital area of weakness or defect in the wall.

Most abdominal hernias are asymptomatic. A hernia is reducible when its contents can be replaced within the surrounding musculature, and it is irreducible or incarcerated when it cannot be reduced. A strangulated hernia has compromised blood supply to its contents, which is a serious and potentially fatal complication. Strangulation occurs more often in large hernias that have small orifices. In this situation, the small neck of the hernia obstructs arterial blood flow, venous drainage, or both to the contents of the hernia sac. Adhesions between the contents of the hernia and peritoneal lining of the sac can provide a tethering point that entraps the hernia contents and predisposes to intestinal obstruction and strangulation. Incarcerated or strangulated hernias cause pain and require immediate surgery.

Rectus diastasis on the other hand is an acquired abdominal wall defect in which the rectus muscles on either side of the midline separate. This is not a true hernia as

O. Ozkaya Mutlu, MD (✉) O. Colak, MD
Division of Plastic, Reconstructive and Aesthetic Surgery,
Okmeydanı Training and Research Hospital,
Istanbul, Turkey
e-mail: ozaydr@gmal.com

M. Atay
General Surgery: Breast Surgery Unit,
Gayrettepe Florence Nightingale Hospital,
Istanbul, Turkey

K.T. Tiryaki (ed.), *Inverse Abdominoplasty*, DOI 10.1007/978-3-319-39310-0_9

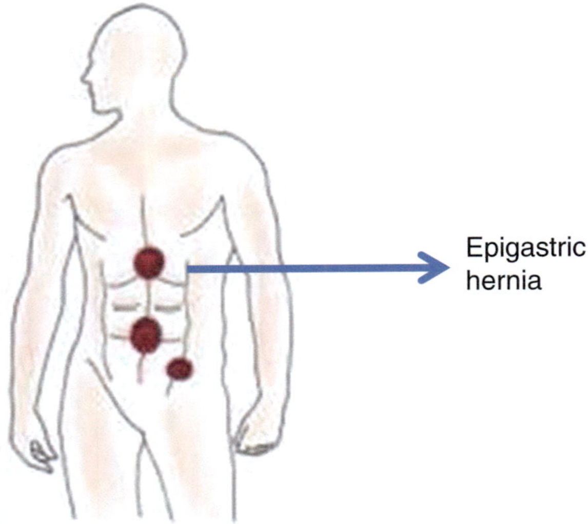

Fig. 9.1 Epigastric hernia

there is no fascial defect, but it is mentioned here for differential diagnosis purposes. Diastasis recti do not create clinical symptoms but might cause aesthetically unpleasant bulging of the abdominal area. Also, pregnancy is a common risk factor [2].

9.2 Classification

Abdominal wall hernias, or external hernias (where abdominal contents protrude beyond the abdominal cavity), include umbilical, epigastric, spigelian, and incisional hernias and eventrations.

9.2.1 Epigastric Hernias

Approximately 3–5 % of the population has epigastric hernias. Epigastric hernias are two to three times more common in men, with the diagnosis usually being made in the third to fifth decades. These hernias occur through the linea alba which is a slight furrow in the midline extending from the ensiform cartilage at the xiphoid process above down to the pubic symphysis below (Fig. 9.1). These are protrusions of properitoneal fat and peritoneum through the decussating fibers of the rectus sheath in the midline. The majority of epigastric hernias (probably 75 %) are asymptomatic. Typical symptoms, if present, include vague upper abdominal pain and nausea associated with epigastric tenderness. The symptoms tend to be more severe when the patient is lying down, attributed to traction on the hernial contents. Pain on exertion localized to the epigastrium is also a common symptom. Although the

Fig. 9.2 Umbilical hernia

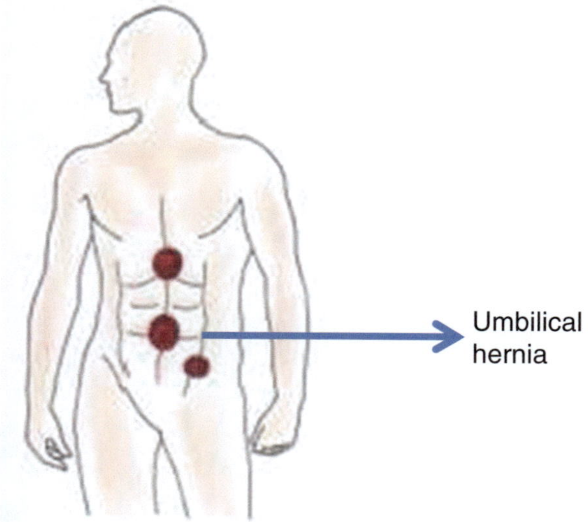

defects are small, they often produce pain out of proportion to their size because of incarceration of preperitoneal fat or omentum. Incarceration or strangulation of the intra-abdominal viscera is extremely rare, with the symptoms obviously depending on the incarcerated organ [1, 3].

9.2.2 Umbilical Hernias

The umbilicus is formed by the umbilical ring of the linea alba. Intra-abdominally, the round ligament (ligamentum teres) and paraumbilical veins join into the umbilicus superiorly, and the median umbilical ligament (obliterated urachus) enters inferiorly. An umbilical hernia traverses the fibromuscular ring of the umbilicus (Fig. 9.2). This hernia is most commonly found in infants and children, is congenital in origin, and often resolves without treatment by the age of five. An acquired umbilical hernia may also be seen in an adult, and this hernia is more common in women with a history of multiple pregnancies and in patients with obesity or with increased abdominal pressure resulting from ascites and chronic bowel distention.

Umbilical hernia is more common in those who have only a single midline aponeurotic decussation compared with the normal decussation of fibers from all three lateral abdominal muscles. Strangulation is unusual in most patients; however, strangulation or rupture can occur in chronic ascitic conditions. Small asymptomatic umbilical hernias barely detectable on examination need not be repaired. Adults who have symptoms, a large hernia, incarceration, thinning of the overlying skin, or uncontrollable ascites should have hernia repair. Spontaneous rupture of umbilical hernias in patients with ascites can result in peritonitis and death [1, 4, 5].

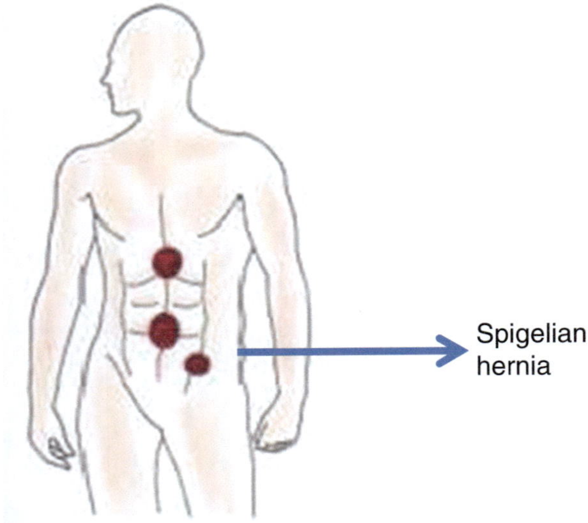

Fig. 9.3 Spigelian hernia

9.2.3 *Spigelian Hernias*

Although spigelian hernias are uncommon (accounting for 0.1–2 % of all abdominal wall hernias), its diagnostic incidence has been rising because of improved imaging technology and incidental identification during laparoscopy. They occur in the anterolateral aspect of the lower abdomen, along the semilunar line formed by fibrous union of the rectus sheath with the aponeuroses of the transversus abdominis and oblique abdominal muscles (Fig. 9.3). The absence of posterior rectus fascia may contribute to an inherent weakness in this area. These hernias are often interparietal, with the hernia sac dissecting posteriorly to the external oblique aponeurosis. Patients usually present with a prolonged history of intermittent lower abdominal pain and intestinal obstruction associated with a slight swelling or vanishing anterolateral mass located midway between the umbilicus and the symphysis pubis. Most spigelian hernias are small (1–2 cm in diameter) and develop during 40–70 years of age, but the hernia has also been reported in younger patients. Spigelian hernias occur with almost equal frequency in males and females; they can be bilateral and associated with other ventral or inguinal hernias. Incarceration rates (often with omentum) have been reported to be as high as 20 % with these uncommon hernias [1, 4–6].

9.2.4 *Incisional Hernias*

Incisional hernias are delayed complications of abdominal surgery and occur in 0.5–13.9 % of patients. These hernias tend to occur during the first four months after surgery, a critical period for the healing of transected muscular and fascial layers of the abdominal wall. Incisional hernias are caused by patient- and surgery-related factors. The former includes conditions that may increase intra-abdominal pressure (e.g., obesity, collagen vascular diseases, a history of surgically repaired aorta, nutritional factors, ascites). Conditions that impair healing, such as collagen vascular disease in patients receiving glucocorticoid therapy and smoking, can also increase postoperative hernia formation. Surgery-related factors include the type and location of the incision. It is more common for hernias to develop after a vertical midline incision than after a transverse incision but to also develop through small laparoscopic puncture sites [4, 7, 8].

9.2.5 Eventration

Regardless of the cause, the loss of integrity of the abdominal wall reduces intra-abdominal pressure and causes serious disturbances, which is appropriately named "eventration disease" by Rives. The salient feature of this syndrome is respiratory dysfunction. A large incisional hernia produces paradoxical respiratory abdominal motion similar to the flail chest. Diaphragmatic function becomes inefficient. The diaphragm no longer contacts against the abdominal viscera and instead forces them into the hernia sac. Appraisal of respiratory function and blood gases is essential [9].

9.3 Preoperative Evaluation of Abdominal Wall Defects

The correct diagnosis of abdominal wall hernias is usually based on careful inspection and palpation; however, there are several situations in which an accurate clinical diagnosis may be difficult or impossible, such as in obese patients, those with severe abdominal pain or distention, and those with excessive scarring. Five to ten percent of abdominal wall hernias are not detectable by physical examination alone [10].

Although most abdominal wall hernias are asymptomatic, they may develop acute complications necessitating emergent surgery. In differential diagnosis it is important to keep in mind that the most challenging misdiagnosed conditions are diastasis recti and abdominal wall tumors [8].

9.3.1 Clinical Evaluation

The evaluation of abdominal wall hernias requires diligent physical examination. The anterior abdominal wall is evaluated with the patient in standing and supine positions, and Valsalva maneuver is also useful to demonstrate the site and size of a hernia. Examination should focus on the umbilicus and any incisions that are present. [1]

9.3.2 Radiological Evaluation

Imaging studies are not required in the normal workup of a hernia. The diagnosis of a hernia was made clinically, with plain radiographs or barium studies in the past. Increasingly, diagnosis is made by CT or ultrasonography.

However, cross-imaging studies may be useful in certain scenarios, as follows:

- If an incarcerated or strangulated wall hernia is suspected, upright abdominal films may be obtained in clinical emergency patients to show small or large bowel obstruction; infrequently, the transition point is seen at the level of the complicated hernia.
- Ultrasonography can be used in differentiating masses in the abdominal wall and allows dynamic evaluation (e.g., during Valsalva maneuver) to confirm herniation of intra-abdominal contents through a wall defect. Ultrasound may also have good specificity and a high positive predictive value for diagnosing postoperative incisional hernias [5, 11].
- Multidetector-row CT (MDCT) is widely available and is fundamental in assessing patients with suspected abdominal wall hernia.
- MDCT or ultrasonography may be necessary if a good examination cannot be obtained because of the patient's body habitus, also mostly to diagnose spigelian hernia [5, 8].

9.3.3 Signs and Symptoms

1. *Characteristics of asymptomatic hernias*:
   - An obvious swelling or fullness beneath the skin at the hernia site
   - A heavy feeling in the abdomen that is sometimes accompanied by constipation
   - Discomfort in the abdomen when lifting or bending over
   - Aching sensation (radiates into the area of the hernia)
   - No true pain or tenderness upon examination
   - Enlarges with increasing intra-abdominal pressure and/or standing
2. *Characteristics of incarcerated hernias*:
   - Painful enlargement of a previous hernia or defect
   - Cannot be manipulated (either spontaneously or manually) through the fascial defect
   - Nausea, vomiting, and symptoms of bowel obstruction (possible)
3. *Characteristics of strangulated hernias*:
   - Patients have symptoms of an incarcerated hernia.
   - Systemic toxicity secondary to ischemic bowel is possible.

- Strangulation is probable if pain and tenderness of an incarcerated hernia persist after reduction.
- Suspect an alternative diagnosis in patients who have a substantial amount of pain without evidence of incarceration or strangulation.

4. *Characteristics of various hernia types*:

- Umbilical hernia – central and mid-abdominal bulge.
- Epigastric hernia – small lumps along the linea alba reflecting openings through which preperitoneal fat can protrude.
- Spigelian hernia – local pain and signs of obstruction from incarceration; pain increases with contraction of the abdominal musculature.

9.4 Treatment of Abdominal Wall Defects

Abdominal wall hernias are either diagnosed on clinical examination or encountered intraoperatively during abdominoplasty. Skin and myofascial laxities, which are often found in overweight, postbariatric or multiparous women, are the primary indications for abdominoplasty procedure (Fig. 9.4). Abdominal

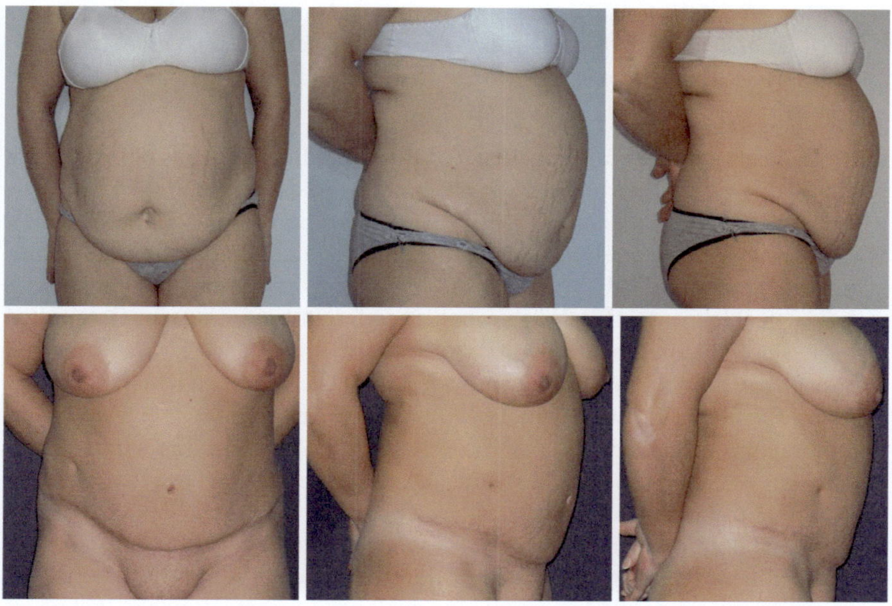

Fig. 9.4 A 44-year-old woman with severe abdominal myofascial laxity and infraumbilical panniculus. In preoperative examination, there was no sign of hernia. Incidental umbilical hernia has been determined in abdominoplasty operation. Above, preoperative views of the patient. Below, postoperative second-year view shows that there is no sign of myofascial laxity

wall hernias are frequently encountered problems associated with the occurrence of fascial laxity or diastasis. Both obesity and pregnancy cause increased intra-abdominal pressure, which are the main causes of rectus diastasis and anterior abdominal wall hernias [12].

It is not uncommon to encounter various degrees of umbilical or paraumbilical incidental hernias during abdominoplasty operations, although symptomatic umbilical hernias can be diagnosed on preoperative physical examination. Also, postbariatric patients have increased risk of incisional hernias with a reported rate of ~20 % [13].

Primary suture techniques, autologous techniques, and placement of prosthetic meshes and bioprosthetics have been described for repair of ventral abdominal hernias.

1. Primary repair

   Incidental hernias during abdominoplasty operations are not rare in clinical practice, although the frequency of incidental hernia in the population and the rate of hernia in abdominoplasty patients are unknown. Usually a primary repair is enough, but first, the separation of the hernia sac from the abdominal wall ring is essential. After the sac is dissected, the peritoneum shall be examined. If intact, simple reduction of the sac is possible, but if the peritoneum is opened or injured, careful dissection and exploration of the intra-abdominal organs (omentum, intestines) is necessary. Following this exploration, the peritoneum should be closed separately. Finally the abdominal wall defect is closed by simple suture technique.

   However, if the fascial defect is larger than 2–3 cm, primary repair techniques are usually inadequate. Synthetic/organic mesh materials are commonly used to bridge the fascial defect with a tension-free closure in such conditions.

2. Synthetic mesh

   Cumberland and Scales popularized the ideal characteristics of prosthetics [14, 15]. These properties include chemical inertness, resistance to mechanical stress, pliability, lack of physical modification by the body's tissues, capability of being sterilized, no carcinogenic potential, no or limited inflammatory or foreign body reaction, and hypoallergenic nature. No prosthetics has been able to attain all these properties so far. In 1958, Usher et al. reported on the newly developed polypropylene mesh (Marlex) which was followed by similar plastic implantable prosthetic materials such as Mersilene and Gore-Tex [16]. This was a notable advance for surgery and allowed tension-free repairs that, when used properly, substantially diminished recurrences after hernia repair procedures. Many abdominal hernias can be repaired using synthetic mesh which lowers the hernia recurrence rates; it is today the first choice in hernia repair (Fig. 9.5). These are associated with serious complications including surgical site infection, extrusion, foreign body reaction, bowel adhesion, fistula formation, and prolonged seroma drainage that occur in ~10–15 % of cases [17, 18]. Infection is one of the most significant causes of recurrent hernia, and the risk of infection is clearly elevated with the risk factors including high body mass index (BMI), smoking status, nutritional

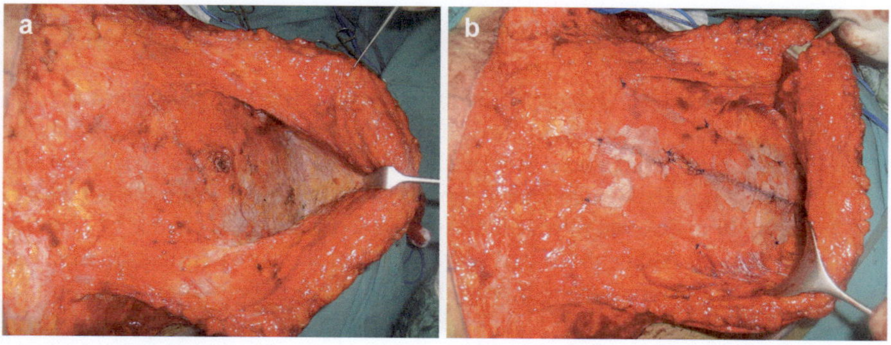

Fig. 9.5 (**a**, **b**) Abdominal wall hernia, primary repair, and inset of the polypropylene mesh

status, steroid treatment, and the presence of comorbidities (e.g., diabetes mellitus, chronic obstructive pulmonary disease (COPD)) in patients who have undergone synthetic mesh placement.

Although synthetic mesh is permanent, the long-term success of these techniques is surprisingly low. Luijendijk et al. in 2000 and Burger et al. in 2004 reported that while mesh is superior to primary suture technique, even mesh repair over a 10-year follow-up period has a 32% failure rate [19, 20].

Removal of previously infected mesh, enterotomies during adhesiolysis, peritonitis, repair of peristomal hernia, open abdominal wall wound, enterocutaneous or enteroatmospheric fistula, and colostomy reversal are commonly accepted contraindications to implantation of synthetic mesh. A relative contraindication is a previous history of infection.

3. Biologic mesh

Biologic mesh is an alternative to synthetic material. Today, there is a shift toward biologic meshes and away from synthetic meshes, particularly in infected or contaminated patients. Ideally, the repair material should be biocompatible or inert, nonallergenic, nonresorbable/permanent, cost-effective, resilient (since no material can be resistant) to infection or contamination, kinematic and having mechanical characteristics with high tensile strength, radiolucent, and accessible for repetitive operative access for intra-abdominal process.

These characteristics are potentially obtainable in many biologic meshes including both allograft and xenograft sources of tissue. Porcine submucosa, human dermis, and porcine dermis are the biologic mesh types that have been reported for ventral hernia repair. Human acellular dermal matrix is a product derived from the human skin and has numerous advantages, including its resistance to infection, the absence of a permanent foreign body at the repair site, and its mechanical properties such as strength to failure, plasticity, and flexibility [21]. Prosthetic repairs are at higher risk for failure in the setting of contamination, colonization, or infection, and thus, autologous reconstruction with flaps or biologic meshes is preferred.

4. Autologous techniques

   (a) Fascia lata graft

      The use of autologous grafts for abdominal hernia repair is not new. In 1932, Gallie [22] reported the use of fascia lata grafts for large abdominal hernia repairs with successful results. McGregor [23] argued that fascia lata was composed of unidirectional proximo-distal fibers which would not remain the multi-directional forces of the anterior abdominal wall created by abdominal contents, although McPeal and Miller [24] supported the use of fascia lata for its minimal foreign body reaction and smooth and glistering surface.

      The tensor fascia lata technique has been described and utilized as a pedicled or free flap, as well as a nonvascularized graft, and has been shown to revascularize, incorporate, and restore peritoneal continuity. As the other autologous tissue-based repairs, this technique has been shown to improve wound healing and outperform traditional synthetic mesh-based techniques in contaminated, tissue-deficient abdominal hernias.

(b)Dermal automesh

The excised dermis in hernia repair during abdominoplasty operations was used by Özkaya Mutlu et al. in 2014 [25]. A standard abdominoplasty operation was performed for all patients who had severe abdominal laxity and type 4 abdomens based on the Matarasso classification system [26]. The long-term results of the use of dermal automesh for the repair of incidental hernias during abdominoplasty operations were evaluated, and a comparative analysis of the biomechanical strengths of dermal automesh vs biological tissue graft was performed in this study (Fig. 9.6). Dermal mesh was compared with FlexHD (which was statistically significantly stronger than other acellular dermal allografts on the market), and although there was no statistically significant difference in tensile strengths, maximum load before yield was found to be ten times higher in dermal automesh than FlexHD's yield power (Fig. 9.7). Long-term clinical and radiologic assessment (anterior abdominal wall MRI studies) of these patients did not show any hernia recurrences.

Reversed dermal grafts had been used in four patients for reconstruction of musculoaponeurotic layer of the anterior abdominal wall and obtained successful results by Costa et al. in 1997 [27]. Kheradmand demonstrated that dermal automesh was readily available in TRAM (Transverse rectus abdominis myocutaneous) flap operations for fascial repair, and its properties meet the criteria for a fascial substitute [28]. However they did not report the biomechanical properties of the dermal tissue. In addition, their follow-up consisted of clinical examination only and no imaging methods. In contrast to these previous studies, Özkaya Mutlu et al. evaluated the biomechanical features of dermal automesh prepared from the panniculus and performed MR studies in long-term follow-up in addition to physical examination (Fig. 9.8). This autograft has several advantages over other techniques such as having durable abdominal wall closure and providing long-term success rates equal to or higher than traditional synthetic mesh-based approaches. Biological materials appear to be less susceptible to infection

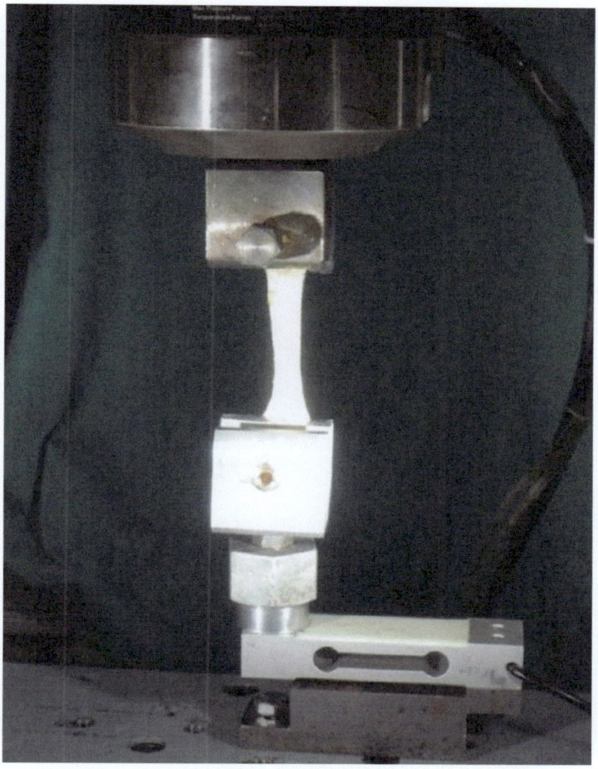

Fig. 9.6 Dog bone-shaped dermal automesh. Uniaxial pulling of the sample by mechanical testing device

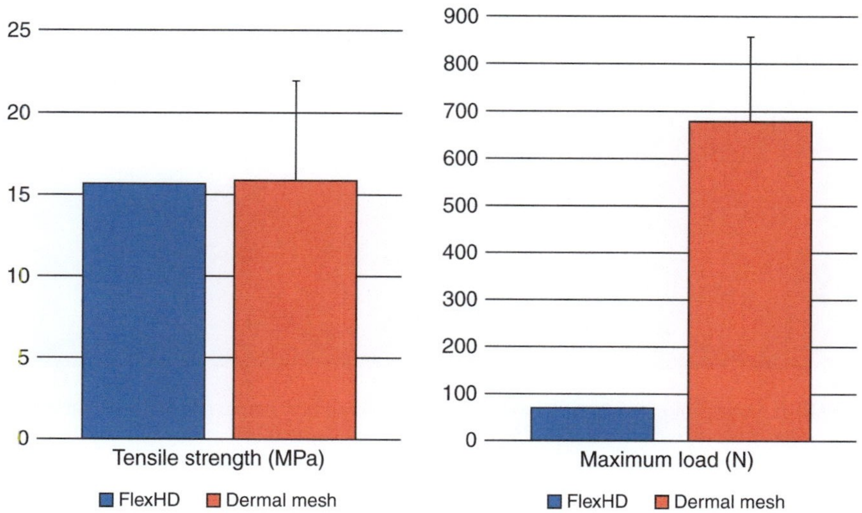

Fig. 9.7 Comparative analysis of tensile strength and maximum lead before yield results of dermal automesh and FlexHD

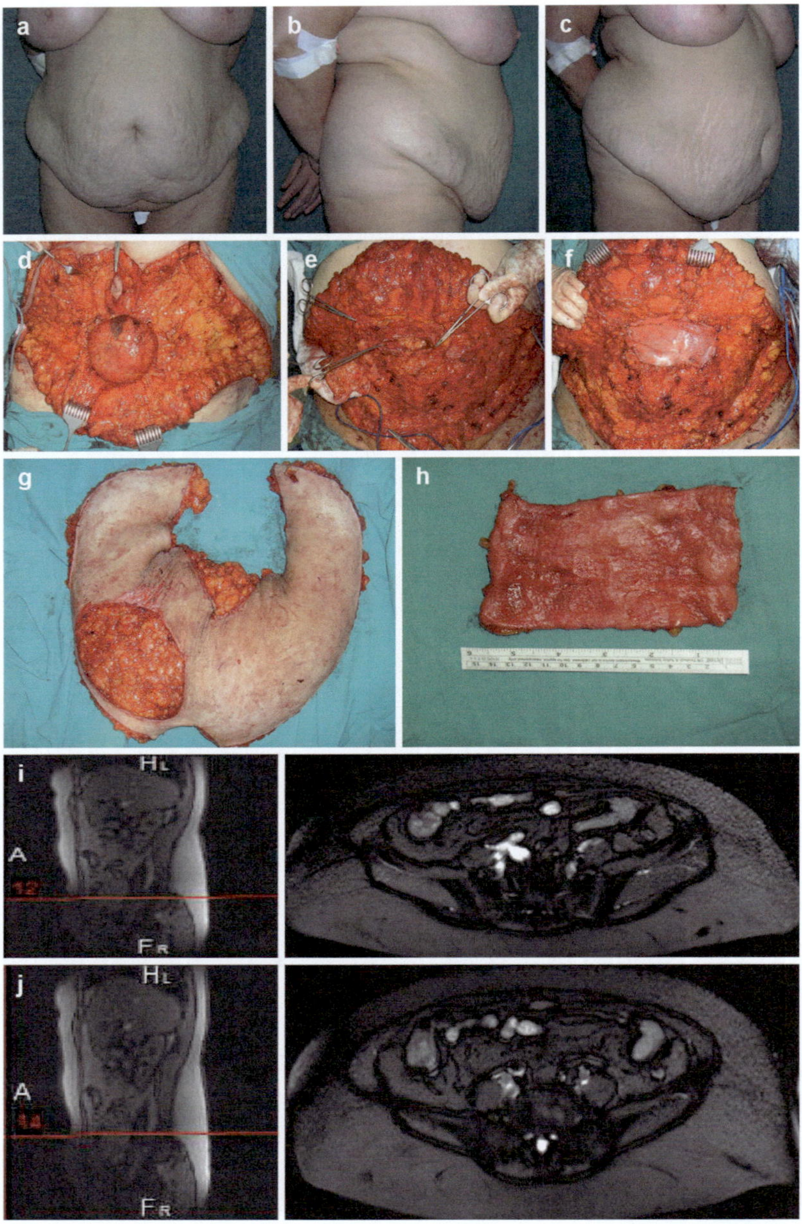

Fig. 9.8 A 44-year-old woman with huge panniculi and umbilical hernia referred from the general surgery department (**a–c**). In the abdominoplasty operation, the hernia was repaired and the dermal automesh was applied to the defect; umbilicus was canceled. Intraoperative view of the hernia (**d**). Umbilicus was canceled and hernia was repaired with primary suture (**e**). The dermal automesh was applied over the repaired area in an onlay fashion (**f**). Preparation of dermal automesh from the panniculus (**g**) Dermal automesh (**h**). Postoperative third-year MRI view shows that there is no recurrence of the hernia (**i**, **j**)

due to rapid vascularization. It was shown that the principal advantages of dermis autografting in TRAM flap donor site closure are ease of use, economy, and the benefit of using an autologous, biological material.

The dermis is a readily available dense fibrous tissue with a high tensile strength, is easy to manipulate, and has limited postoperative absorption. Dermal automesh possesses all the positive properties of the acellular cadaveric dermis with the added benefit of sufficient tensile strength, cost-effectivity, easy availability in the operation room, and the lack of any added morbidity, which correlates with the fact that dermal automesh becomes revascularized in situ. This autograft can be used to avoid the possible complications of synthetic materials in patients who are noted to have an incidental hernia during abdominoplasty. Onlay use of the dermal automesh prepared from the excised panniculus after tension-free primary repair of hernias that are not very wide and are clinically asymptomatic decreases hernia recurrences and eliminates the complications associated with the use of synthetic mesh materials (Fig. 9.9).

According to experiences of Özkaya Mutlu et al., dermal automesh can be used in small- and medium-sized hernia repair safely. For larger hernias, further assessment is necessary. The authors did not have any mesh-related complications, like infection, delayed wound healing, extrusion, and fistula formation, which are significant problems for permanent materials. The tensile strength of the dermal mesh is resistant enough to intra-abdominal pressure for avoiding any hernia recurrence. The lack of the need for extra material and cost-effectivity are the other advantages of this technique (Table 9.1).

Umbilical Hernias

The separation of the hernia sac from the umbilical ring is essential during surgery. Once the sac is separated, the peritoneum is examined. If it is intact, simple reduction of the sac is possible, but if the peritoneum is opened or injured, careful dissection of the sac and the exploration of the intra-abdominal organs (omentum, intestines) afterward are necessary. Following this exploration, the peritoneum should be closed separately.

After exposure of the umbilical sac, a plane is created to encircle the sac at the level of the fascial ring, and the defect is closed by simple or vest-over-pants suture technique (Fig. 9.10). Defects larger than 3 cm are closed using prosthetic mesh. The mesh might be placed under or over the fascia.

9.4.1 Epigastric Hernias

The hernia and its contents are dissected free of the surrounding tissues and, if present, the hernial contents examined and dealt with appropriately. If the defect is small (2 cm), repair by primary suture closure using nonabsorbable material is usually sufficient. If the defect is large (6 cm^2) or occurs within a divarication of the recti, the hernia should be repaired with mesh. Intermediate-sized hernias are controversial and suture or mesh techniques are both currently acceptable [3].

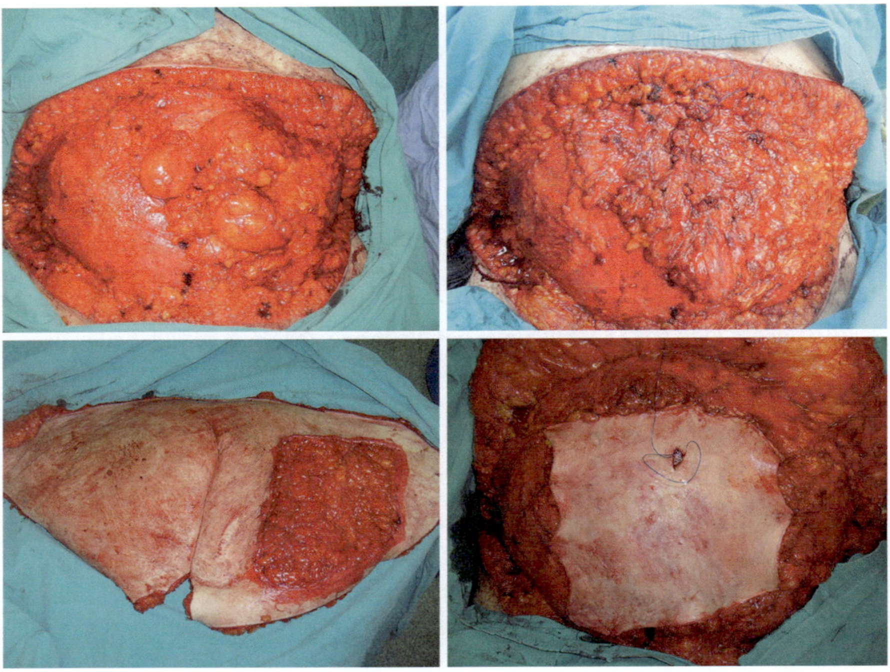

Fig. 9.9 A 46-year-old woman underwent abdominoplasty operation. After flap elevation, a para-umbilical hernia was encountered. All of the hernia contents were reduced and defect was sutured in primary fashion. Then dermal automesh was prepared accordingly and sutured in onlay fashion on the suture line and the weak parts of the abdomen

Table 9.1 Advantages and disadvantages of dermal automesh

Dermal automesh	
Advantages	Disadvantages
Small- and medium-sized hernia repair	No available data for hernias >10 cm
Available in operation	Thickness depends on preparation
Cost-effectivity	Preparation time takes approximately 30 min
Without synthetic mesh complications	
Tensile strength	

9.4.2 Spigelian Hernias

A transverse incision is made over the hernia to the sac. The anterior rectus sheath is incised transversely, and the sac is dissected as far as its neck and either excised or inverted (Fig. 9.11). If the defect is small, it can be closed by simple anatomical repair with a continuous suture of nonabsorbable material. Alternatively, a mesh may be placed in the large defect and sutured to the edges of the defect. Laparoscopic methods are increasingly being employed to repair spigelian hernias.

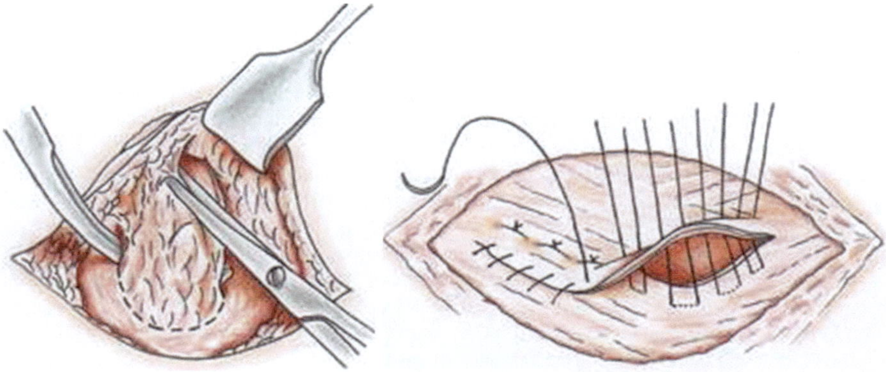

Fig. 9.10 Repair of umbilical hernia

Fig. 9.11 Repair of spigelian hernia

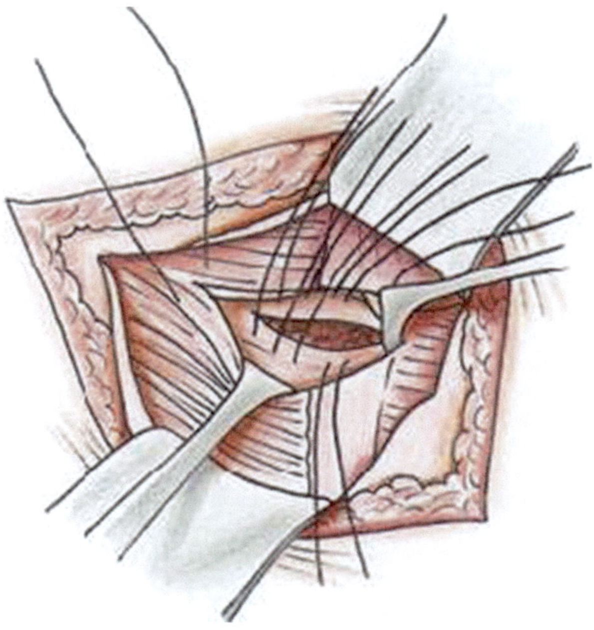

9.4.3 *Incisional Hernias*

Primary repair of incisional hernias can be done when the defect is small (≤2–3 cm in diameter), and there is viable surrounding tissue. Larger defects (>2–3 cm in diameter) have a high recurrence rate if closed primarily and are repaired with a mesh [29]. Recurrence rates vary between 10 and 50 % and are typically reduced by more than 50 % with the use of mesh [1, 30].

References

1. Malangoni MA, Rosen MJ. Hernias. In: Townsend CM, Daniel Beauchamp Jr R, Mark Evers B, Mattox KL, editors. Sabiston textbook of surgery. 19th ed. Philadelphia: E Saunders; 2012. p. 1114–40.
2. Lentz GM. Anatomic defects of the abdominal wall and pelvic floor. In: Lentz GM, Lobo RA, Gershenson DM, Katz VL, editors. Comprehensive gynecology. 6th ed. Philadelphia: E Mosby; 2012. p. 453–74.
3. de Beaux AC. Abdominal hernias. In: Paterson-Brown S, editor. Core topics in general & emergency surgery: companion to specialist surgical. 5th ed. Philadelphia: E Saunders; 2014. p. 57–80.
4. Gore RM, Ghahremani GG, Donaldson CK, Marn CS. Hernias and abdominal wall pathology. In: Gore RM, Levine MS, editors. Textbook of gastrointestinal radiology. 4th ed. Philadelphia: E Saunders; 2015. p. 2053–76.
5. Fitch MT, Manthey DE. Abdominal hernia reduction. In: Roberts JR, Hedges JR, editors. Roberts and Hedges' clinical procedures in emergency medicine. 6th ed. Philadelphia: E Saunders; 2014. p. 873–9.
6. Blatnik JA, Rosen MJ. Ventral herniation in adults. In: Yeo CJ, McFadden DW, Pemberton JH, Peters JH, Matthews JB, editors. Shackelford's surgery of the alimentary tract. 7th ed. Philadelphia: E Saunders; 2012. p. 597–612.
7. Dunbar KB, Rohan Jeyarajah D. Abdominal hernias and gastric volvulus. In: Feldman M, Friedman LS, Brandt LJ, editors. Sleisenger and Fordtran's gastrointestinal and liver disease. 10th ed. Philadelphia: E Saunders; 2016. p. 407–25.
8. Aguirre DA, Rivero OM, Martinez J. Abdominal wall hernias. In: Sahani D, Samir A, editors. Abdominal imaging. Philadelphia: E Saunders; 2011. p. 1464–77.
9. Seymour NE, Bell RE. Abdominal Wall, Omentum, Mesentery, and Retroperitoneum. In: Brunicardi FC, Andersen DK, Billiar TR, Dunn DL, Hunter JG, Matthews JB, Pallock RE, editors. Schwartz's Principles of Surgery. 9th ed. New York: McGraw-Hill Professional; 2009. p. 1267–82.
10. Lee GH, Cohen AJ. CT imaging of abdominal hernias. AJR Am J Roentgenol. 1993;161:1209–13.
11. den Hartog D, Dur AH, Kamphuis AG, et al. Comparison of ultrasonography with computed tomography in the diagnosis of incisional hernias. Hernia. 2009;13:45–8.
12. Regnault P. Abdominoplasty by the W technique. Plast Reconstr Surg. 1975;55:265.
13. Shermak MA. Hernia repair and abdominoplasty in gastric bypass patients. Plast Reconstr Surg. 2006;117:1145–50.
14. Cumberland VH. A preliminary report on the use of prefabricated nylon weave in the repair of ventral hernia. Med J Aust. 1952;1:143.
15. Scales JT. Tissue reactions to synthetic materials. Proc R Soc Med. 1953;46:647.
16. Usher FC, Ochsner J, Tuttle Jr LL. Use of marlex mesh in the repair of incisional hernias. Am Surg. 1958;24:969.
17. Bauer JJ, Harris MT, Kreel I, et al. Twelve-year experience with expanded polytetrafluoroethylene in the repair of abdominal wall defects. Mt Sinai J Med. 1999;66:20–5.
18. Trupka AW, Schweiberer L, Hallfeldt K, et al. Management of large abdominal wall hernias with foreign implant materials (Gore-Tex patch). Zentralbl Chir. 1997;122:879–84.
19. Luijendijk RW, Hop WC, van den Tol MP, et al. A comparison of suture repair with mesh repair for incisional hernia. N Engl J Med. 2000;343:392.
20. Burger JW, Luijendijk RW, Hop WC, et al. Long term follow up of a randomized controlled trial of suture versus mesh repair of incisional hernia. Ann Surg. 2004;240:578–83.
21. Silverman RP, Li EN, Holton 3rd LH, et al. Ventral hernia repair using allogenic acellular dermal matrix in a swine model. Hernia. 2004;8:336–42.
22. Gallie WE. Closing very large hernial openings. Ann Surg. 1932;96:551–5.

23. McGregor IA. The use of dermis to reconstruct the musculo- aponeurotic element of the anterior abdominal wall. Br J Plast Surg. 1991;44:619–21.
24. McPeal CJ, Miller R. Abdominal wall replacement. Surgery. 1960;47:944–8.
25. Ozkaya Mutlu O, Egemen O, Akan A, et al. The use of dermal automesh for incidental hernia repair in abdominoplasty: clinical, biochemical, and radiological results. J Plast Surg Hand Surg. 2014;49:1–5.
26. Matarasso A. Abdominoplasty. Clin Plast Surg. 1989;16:289.
27. Costa H, Cunha C, Conde A, et al. The reversed dermal graft concept in abdominal wall reconstruction. Eur J Plast Surg. 1997;20:186–91.
28. Kheradmand AA, Novin NR, Khazaeipour Z. Brief report: the use of dermal autograft for fascial repair of TRAM flap donor sites. J Plast Reconstr Aesthet Surg. 2011;64:364–8.
29. Wright BE, Beckerman J, Cohen M. Is laparoscopic umbilical hernia repair with mesh a reasonable alternative to conventional repair? Am J Surg. 2002;184:505–8; discussion 508–509.
30. Anthony T, Bergen PC, Kim LT, et al. Factors affecting recurrence following incisional herniorrhaphy. World J Surg. 2000;24:95–100.

Chapter 10
Prevention and Management of Abdominoplasty Complications

Semih Baghaki and Lina Triana

10.1 Introduction

Abdominoplasty is performed to shape the anterior and lateral abdominal walls. Different forms of contour deformity should be addressed with modifications and combinations of techniques. Either traditional abdominoplasty or high-lateral-tension abdominoplasty (HLTA) is usually combined with liposuction of the anterior abdominal wall and love handles giving satisfactory results most of the time. Although this combination covers a good percentage of patients complaining of lower abdominal sagging or bulging, some other techniques are also present such as mini abdominoplasty, fleur-de-lis abdominoplasty, and reverse abdominoplasty. Post bariatric patients need further ablative procedures such as dermolipectomy and belt lipectomy.

Besides being a rewarding surgery, abdominoplasty harbors a spectrum of cosmetic and non-cosmetic complications. By definition, abdominoplasty is considered to have the highest complication rate among aesthetic surgical procedures [1]. In order to decrease the complication rate and increase cosmetic results together with patient satisfaction, every single step of diagnosis and treatment should be controlled and tailored according to the needs and characteristics of each patient. Patient selection, operative design, surgical technique, and postoperative care should be detailed in order to minimize complications.

S. Baghaki
Department of Plastic and Reconstructive Surgery, Istanbul University, Cerrahpasa Medical Faculty, Cali, Colombia

L. Triana (✉)
Corpus and Rostrum Surgery Center, Cali, Colombia
e-mail: linatriana@drlinatriana.com

K.T. Tiryaki (ed.), *Inverse Abdominoplasty*, DOI 10.1007/978-3-319-39310-0_10

10.2 Preoperative Evaluation, Indications, and Contraindications

Most of the patients seeking abdominal contouring have some common features. These can be summarized as being unable to sustain a stable weight and conditioning and having history of pregnancy, massive weight changes, or abdominal surgery and some degree of abdominal wall laxity. Patients may or may not be obese. Besides these patients, a number of relatively fit patients also admit to have lower abdominal contouring in order to improve appearance.

In order to avoid major complications and patient dissatisfaction, patients should be elected according to some factors. One of the most important factors is to distinguish body habitus and either to disqualify patients having centripedal obesity or plan to operate on those patients in a staged manner, i.e., sequential high-lateral-tension abdominoplasty (HLTA) and reverse abdominoplasty or HLTA and liposuction. These patients have intra-abdominal visceral fat accumulation. This chronic process results in tissue expansion of the anterior abdominal wall with thinning of the fascial and muscular layers. Such a chronic biomechanical change cannot be reversed acutely in a 2-h operation addressing only the skin, superficial fascial system, and anterior rectus sheath. The body mass indices (BMI) of these patients are usually above 30, although rarely it can be between 25 and 30.

It is very important during consultation to physically show to the patient the intra-abdominal visceral fat accumulation if present so that they understand why the chosen surgical procedure will not leave them with a totally flat abdomen. The easiest way to do this is to put the patient in a sideways standing position in front of a mirror and grasp with a pinch maneuver the amount of superficial fat present (fat above the Scarpa fascia). The amount of abdomen protrusion seen after isolating this superficial fat in the pinch maneuver stands for the amount of abdomen muscle diastasis and intra-abdominal visceral fat present.

A history of rapid weight changes also indicates either uncontrolled diet and lifestyle or a metabolic predisposition due to dysregulated adipokine trafficking [2, 3]. Patients should be in the same weight range of +/− 10 pounds for a year. This range should be interpreted according to the ethnic and demographic factors of population. Like any other surgical procedure, patient should be cleared of uncontrolled comorbidities, such as hypertension, coronary artery disease, diabetes mellitus, vasculitides, and chronic use of medications or herbal adjuncts. Smoking has long been considered as a relative contraindication, and the patient should quit smoking at least 3–4 weeks before the operation. Excessive alcohol consumption might increase bleeding time especially with the use of nonsteroidal anti-inflammatory drugs.

A thorough physical examination should be performed. Abdominal scars which may compromise skin flap viability, e.g., subcostal or paramedian incisions, are noted. Diastasis recti and possible ventral hernias should be ruled out by physical examination in the upright and supine position, with and without Valsalva maneuver. In overweight or obese patients, hernias can be difficult to palpate. Although physical examination is usually enough to detect fascial dehiscence and most of the hernias, ultrasound examination should also be used for confirmation when needed.

10.3 Informing the Patient

Preoperative informing of the patient is crucial as always in aesthetic plastic surgery. The level of perception of a patient is totally different before and after the operation. Every aspect of the operation including length and height of the scars, amount of narrowing of waistline, functional layoff, change in umbilicus, and potential complications should be explained in detail. Surgical revisions might take place and should be told before abdominoplasty. Especially combined procedures, e.g., breast reduction plus abdominoplasty and thigh lift plus abdominoplasty, increase the incidence of complications and length of recovery.

10.4 Preoperative Preparation

The patient should adjust bowel habits to a more liquid diet to prevent constipation. Increased intra-abdominal pressure constitutes difficulty to close abdominal flap during surgery and also causes discomfort postoperatively. Some surgeons prefer to clean bowel with an enema the night before the operation. The patient should urinate before surgery to prevent a distended bladder resulting in increased intra-abdominal volume. This also might avoid the need for urinary catheter which can be a source of bacteremia in patients with obesity and/or diabetes [4]. The patient should discontinue smoking for at least 2–3 weeks before and 2–3 weeks after surgery. High-risk patients for deep vein thrombosis (DVT) should be given low-molecular-weight heparin 12 h prior to surgery and continued according to the Caprini scale scorings. Compression garments should be worn by the patient before surgery as well [5].

10.5 Postoperative Care

Postoperative period of abdominoplasty is usually straightforward with early mobilization, removal of drains in 2–3 days, and limited physical activity during the first 2 weeks. The patient is placed in bed with the head, knees, and feet elevated. Liquid diet is started and then advanced. Although subfascial infiltration of local anesthetics is useful, narcotic analgesics or a pain pump can be used for postoperative analgesia. Patient should be mobilized as early as possible. Compression garments or devices should be used until full ambulation is obtained. Patients should be walking slightly flexed at the waist for a few days. Although abdominal binders do not offer physical advantage for mobilization, they give a feeling of safety while walking. The abdominal binder is kept on for the first week, and it should not be so tight since increased intra-abdominal pressure increases the risk of thromboembolic complications.

Intermittent leg compression garments should be used until the patient is able to get out of bed. The use of compression socks for 10–20 days after surgery is also advisable.

Showering is allowed two days after the operation regardless if drains are in place. Since it takes some time to regain cutaneous sensation of the abdominal wall, patients are instructed not to apply heating pads to the abdomen or sunbathe. Driving is allowed whenever patient feels comfortable. Abdominal muscle exercises can be started after 4–6 weeks. Strenuous physical activities should be prohibited for 6 weeks. Patient should be informed that early ecchymoses and edema resolve in 2–3 weeks.

10.6 Main Complications of Abdominoplasty

Abdominoplasty is an extensive operation with potential risks and complications that need to be considered by both the patient and plastic surgeon. Abdominoplasty, which is usually combined with some extent of liposuction, carries arguably the highest complication rate among aesthetic surgery procedures. As a general rule, complications are more common in higher-BMI patients, and many patients that present for abdominoplasty are in the overweight-to-obese range [6]. Potential complications of abdominoplasty are discussed below.

10.6.1 Aesthetic Complications

10.6.1.1 Place and Quality of Abdominal Scar

Residual scar after abdominoplasty can be relatively long or highly leveled. Complaints on resultant scar can be exaggerated despite the scar being actually fairly well. Most of the time, this results from inadequate preoperative informing of the patient or selecting a patient with high expectations who does not accept mentioned possible surgical results. If the patient is cooperating with the surgeon during preoperative period and understands the needs of her body habitus, most of the time, a longer incision shaping the abdomen, flanks, and inguinal areas well enough is welcomed.

Asymmetric abdominal scar is another aesthetic complication almost always resulting from inadequate preoperative planning and intraoperative tailoring. Correction of dog ears should be performed with utmost precision. This can be accomplished with liberal use of liposuction laterally and excision of redundant skin step by step comparing both sides [7]. This is especially important in high-lateral-tension abdominoplasty where lateral excision is fundamental. This outcome is usually caused by a poor marking design with either an overestimation or under-estimation skin redundancy below the incision. If there is significant excess below the incision, the resultant scar might be high riding. If there is no excessive redundant skin below the incision, the scar might be too low if too much skin is excised. As always in plastic surgery, the remaining volume is more important than the resected volume. Thus, remaining skin flaps must ensure a final scar shortly above the anterior superior iliac spinae. If the technique used is high-lateral-tension abdominoplasty, then some degree of thigh lift will be provided, and the final scar will be a longer one extending laterally above the anterior superior iliac spinae. Most of the patients, if the scar is thin enough and the operation gives good shaping of the flank and thigh areas, do not complain much about the length of the scar. Prevention of dog ears is a must during closure since, although the length of the scar is not a major patient complaint as described before; any skin excess especially in the lateral aspects of the scar can potentially end up with an unhappy patient.

10.6.1.2 Change in the Position of Pubic Area

One of the main reasons for a patient seeking abdominoplasty is ptotic mons. Abdominoplasty should also correct the position of the mons pubis at least to some degree. Placing the incision so close to the symphysis pubis, which is closer than 6 cm, results in a stretched and heightened pubis. Besides being a cosmetic deformity, this might lead to localized lymphedema of the area which may not resolve in long time. To place the incision too far from the symphysis pubis, which is further than 8 cm, avoids significant shaping of the pubis resulting in redundant pubic skin and soft tissues. Liposuction of the pubic area is a critical procedure which should be reserved for a very few number of patients. Besides being seemingly straightforward, overtreatment of this area with liposuction might result in permanent lymphedema and/or neurovascular damage of the clitoris. If any residual volume problems of the pubic area exist after abdominoplasty, this can be addressed with secondary partial excisions, limited liposuctions, and/or fat injections. In patients who have a highly positioned umbilicus, the mons pubis can migrate superiorly with closure of abdominal flap. This potential complication can be prevented by closing umbilical defect with a purse string suture or a T-shaped scar which may end up like a fleur-de-lis scar.

The quality of scar can be questioned by the patient. Patients should always remember that as plastic surgeons we cannot predict 100 % how a final scar will appear. This is very important to be addressed to the patient before the surgery since the final quality of the scar is multifactorial and includes endogenous patient conditions, surgeon´s operative techniques, and patient aftercare. Bad scars can be either hypertrophic or atrophic. Preoperatively, the patient should be questioned and examined about the quality of previous scars, if present. A history of hypertrophic scar or keloid is predictive of the quality of central transverse scar after abdominoplasty. Widened atrophic scars can be seen in patients with Caucasian origin. Atrophic scars are often the result of inadequate reapproximation of the superficial fascial system. The final status of a scar can be determined at 1 year postoperatively, and bad scars can be revised thereafter. Steroid injections often help to soften hypertrophic scars. Ablative laser procedures can also improve cosmetic result of a hypertrophic scar [8]. Keloids should be addressed with core excision combined with steroid injections.

10.6.1.3 Contour Irregularity

High-lateral-tension abdominoplasty (HLTA) is quite a different operation than traditional abdominoplasty. In the latter, the resection is aimed mainly to lower midline redundancy between the umbilicus and the pubis, whereas in HLTA the excess is considered more in lateral than in the midline. This mainly lateral excision results in more lift in the anterolateral thigh. Still, some contour problems may persist after either traditional abdominoplasty or HLTA.

Epigastric and/or hypogastric bulging is one of the most annoying problems after abdominoplasty. This may result from inadequate plication of the supraumbilical rectus sheath or more commonly from picking the wrong patient for abdominoplasty. An epigastric bulge is usually indicative of voluminous omental fat, and these patients are best treated after a vigorous period of weight loss and physical exercise. Although HLTA has a superolateral vector of pull and can shape this redundancy, the patient with significant epigastric bulging should be informed preoperatively that this problem may persist. A fleur-de-lis or reverse abdominoplasty can better treat this problem and should be offered to patient either primarily or secondarily.

Central or infraumbilical bulging results from either insufficient thinning of central abdominoplasty flap or inadequate plication of the rectus sheath at this segment. Although it is an attempt with good will with the belief that a thicker flap will be perfused better, any remaining fat under the Scarpa fascia does not provide perfusion advantage to this area [9]. Preservation of subcostal perforators during elevation of abdominoplasty flap will enable surgeon to effectively perform liposuction and prepare a thin enough flap with adequate perfusion.

Lateral dog ears are another well-known problem after abdominoplasty. Although small dog ears improve over time, it is best to address this problem intraoperatively. To decrease the incidence and magnitude of this problem, lateral liposuction should be liberally used followed by careful excision of redundant skin with precise measuring and comparison bilaterally extending laterally as much as needed [10]. While closing whole abdominal incision, symmetric stay sutures can be placed to advance superior flap medially from both sides. This usually creates a harmonic lateral contour and primary closure can be started from the lateral to medial. In my personal experience, in patients with good dermal thickness, lateral ends of the abdominal incision can be closed with purse string sutures. This type of closure decreases the length of incision and lifts up the groin and thigh in selected cases.

10.6.1.4 Umbilical Problems

Preparation and placement of umbilicus need careful surgical skills. Preoperative marking of the umbilicus is important for appropriate dissection and shaping. Umbilical malposition or deformity can occur after abdominoplasty and can be avoided with careful preoperative marking. Previous abdominal operations should be questioned and the location of scars should be noted. Especially laparoscopic operations almost always use umbilical trocar, and it is not uncommon to observe some degree of fascial dehiscence at the umbilical stalk. This might both lead to inadequate shaping and late-term migration of the umbilicus.

Bad scarring of the umbilicus is a rare but disturbing complication due to either poor skin quality or surgical technique. Closing under tension, placement of dermal sutures superficially and inappropriate preoperative marking are main reasons for this complication. Secondary corrections might be needed if watchful waiting or a single dose of steroid injection does not work.

10.6.2 Physiologic Complications

10.6.2.1 Hematoma

Hematoma is one of the potential complications of abdominoplasty. This complication usually occurs in the first two days of the operation. Close monitoring of blood pressure and heart rate is fundamental during the first day of the operation if the patient is not discharged. Increase in heart rate together with steady decrease in blood pressure is indicative of hematoma unless proved otherwise. If a hematoma advances, clinical symptoms such as feeling of abdominal pressure and pain are observed. Clinically evident hematomas are usually accompanied with tachycardia and some degree of hypotension necessitating drainage, exploration, and hemostasis. After surgical hemostasis, abdominal flap may suffer some degree of necrosis either superficial or full thickness due to ischemia reperfusion injury. Limited hematomas can be managed conservatively, unless they cause hemodynamic changes.

In order to decrease the rate of this complication, there are some points to be considered. For instance, preoperatively the patient should be questioned about the medical history in detail. A history of hypertension, current use of herbal adjuncts causing antiaggregant effect such as green tea, history of easy bruising, history of prolonged bleeding after dental procedures, current use of medications causing prolongation in bleeding time such as nonsteroidal anti-inflammatory drugs, and current use of alcohol beyond social levels give enough idea about the possibility of hematoma formation. Preoperatively, liberal use of cautery does not mean that this will prevent hematoma formation. Indeed, dissection with cautery without isolation of perforators results in immediate contraction of perforators especially the ones along the rectus sheath. If these vessels cannot be coagulated in the first attempt and then got underneath the rectus sheath, fascia should be opened, and hemostasis should be achieved with bipolar cautery since they are hard to catch. In the first sight, they may seem to be coagulated, but with the completion of operation and increase in blood pressure, it is pretty possible that these vessels can open up. Therefore, the best technique is using perforator flap dissection techniques where a pair of Metzenbaum scissors and an Adson forceps without teeth are used. Perforators especially those of rectus muscle in origin should be skeletonized first without disruption and then coagulated with the use of bipolar cautery. Other perforators such as lateral intercostal, subcostal, and lumbar ones should always be preserved during flap elevation. This approach will also prevent the formation of hematoma inside the rectus sheath which can be life threatening unless treated immediately. Hemostatic clips can also be used to ligate these vessels. Control of blood pressure is of crucial importance during early postoperative period. Abdominal binders, although widely used, do not guarantee prevention of hematoma formation.

10.6.2.2 Seroma

The most frequent complication of abdominoplasty is the formation of seroma. This is usually the result of extensive undermining and/or liberal use of monopolar cautery during the operation although the etiology is not completely understood. Limited use of monopolar cautery seems to decrease serous discharge after the operation, although this may not translate into rate of seroma formation [11–13]. Jackson-Pratt drains almost always are enough to drain collections. Abdominal binders are believed to decrease the rate of this complication although this is not evidence based. Adherence of the abdominal flap to the underlying abdominal wall is important to prevent seroma formation. Obliterating dead spaces with quilting mattress sutures is a widely used technique to adhere abdominal flap to the deep fascia.

If a seroma forms and persist after a week or two, repeated aspirations and even reinsertion of a closed suction drain is required. If seroma still persists surgical exploration, excision of the seroma capsule might be needed. Excision or capsulotomy should be followed with quilting sutures to obliterate the dead space. Low-volume seromas tend to resolve without any therapy from a few weeks to a few months. In my personal practice, I almost always perform HLTA with the use of knife and scissors then combine with liposuction and choose patients suitable for this technique. This results in drain removal in the first 24 h of operation. Because of the less dissection character of HLTA, I have observed no clinically evident seromas to date. Preserving epifascial lymphatic network is another trick that may help avoiding seroma formation most probably due to improved contact of like tissues between abdominal flap and adipofascial tissues overlying deep fascia of the anterior abdominal wall [14]. Despite all discussion and different approaches, surgeon may very well perform abdominoplasty with immense thinning of abdominal flap without preserving the Scarpa fascia.

This can be combined with limited delamination where quilting sutures can be omitted even together with drains [15, 16].

10.6.2.3 Delayed Wound Healing

Delayed wound healing and dehiscence can be seen after abdominoplasty. Predisposing factors are not difficult to guess. These include history of smoking, presence of upper abdominal scars, closure under excessive tension, and undrained hematomas. Operating on high-risk patients such as diabetics and smokers is obviously not a good idea since wound healing problems are disturbing, time wasting, and socially isolating. Therefore "preconditioning of the patient" by cessation of smoking and strict control of metabolic imbalances are of paramount importance. From a technical point of view, extensive delamination, aggressive liposuction of abdominal skin and soft tissues, and excessive thinning of central lower abdominal flap in an attempt to resect as much skin as possible usually end up with some degree of healing problems or at least low quality of life during early postoperative period.

Wound dehiscence after abdominoplasty can arise due to inadequate closure of the superficial fascial system or uncontrolled extension of the trunk during early postoperative period. The patient should keep her position flexed at the waist for at least 4–5 days after surgery and be cautious while getting up from bed. Postoperative necrosis or dehiscence of abdominal flap is treated with a period of wound care and delayed primary closure. Most of these patients require 4–6 weeks in order to have their wound ready to be closed. During wound care period, detailed gauze debridement should be performed inside the cavity. Antiseptic solutions or irrigation with normal saline does not benefit without meticulous sterile examination, gauze debridement, and wet-to-dry dressings of the cavity. If the patient is going to be followed in the hospital, vacuum-assisted closure systems should be used in order to decrease hospital stay and decrease labor [17].

Wound infections can present in the form of cellulitis of the anterior abdominal wall and/or an infected hematoma/seroma. Cellulitis has a definitive clinical picture composed of active hyperemia, tenderness (pain with palpation), swelling, and peau d'orange appearance. Uncomplicated cellulitis can easily be treated with systemic (either oral or parenteral) and topical antibiotics. If any degree of detachment or epithelialization defect has been observed, the incision should be opened, and active wound care should be commenced. Most of the time, the surgeon observes only serous discharge and a decrease in level of pain after drainage without purulent discharge or abscess formation. In patients with predisposition such as diabetics or smokers, localized wound infections can evolve into systemic inflammatory response syndrome (SIRS) and, if not detected and treated, into sepsis. Any septic signs such as malaise, nausea, and loss of appetite should be taken seriously with or without fever. Treatment should be started urgently, and this includes drainage, open wound care, systemic antibiotics, intravenous hydration and transfusion of fresh frozen plasma, and/or erythrocyte suspensions as necessary. Surgical drainage should not be delayed for any workup or consultation if such a septic wound infection is suspected.

10.6.2.4 Paresthesia

Some patients might complain of numbness in the central lower abdominal area. This problem decreases with time in majority of patients. If it persists, this manifests as sharp painful points rather than dull painful areas. Patients with persistent paresthesia or pain in the lower abdomen should be cleared with gastrointestinal and gynecologic workup. Injections of local anesthetics combined with low-potent steroids and adrenaline relieve symptoms. These injections can be repeated as needed to break pain circle.

10.6.2.5 Deep Venous Thrombosis and Pulmonary Embolism

Pulmonary embolism (PE) is a rare but life-threatening complication of abdominoplasty. Abdominoplasty when combined with other procedures increases thromboembolism risk from 0.2 to 9.3 % [18].

The increased intra-abdominal pressure caused by abdominal wall plication has been implicated as the cause of decreased venous return from the lower extremity back into the pelvis, thus leading to an increased risk of DVT and pulmonary embolism. Any patient who has shortness of breath or chest pain in the postoperative period should be examined and cleared for pulmonary embolism.

In an aim to decrease thromboembolism appearance, it is advisable to use the Caprini scale scoring in all patients undergoing abdominoplasties; with it, correct thromboprophylaxis can be applied to each individual patient.

Early ambulation in a few hours after the operation is probably the best method to reduce the risk of DVT and PE. There are some other important points to be taken into consideration. For instance, compression garments should be used before transfer to the operating room until the patient starts walking. Oral contraceptives (OCs) have been shown to increase thromboembolic events. Patients using oral contraceptives are either not accepted for abdominoplasty or should quit using these for a cycle before the operation. Smokers are also under higher risk of thromboembolic events, and it is best to either avoid smokers or have them stop it 3–4 weeks before abdominoplasty. Patients should be examined for subclinical deep venous insufficiency with clinical examination and, if needed, with Doppler ultrasound. Low-molecular-weight heparin can be used before and after the operation with a small risk of hematoma. Especially in high-risk patients, i.e., smokers, patients using OCs, and patients with a history of previous embolic events and suspected or proven venous insufficiency of lower extremities (including heavy varicose veins), low-molecular-weight heparin should be used. Heparinization should be accompanied with strict control of blood pressure avoiding hypertension. During early postoperative period, any patient having chest pain, difficulty in breathing, calf pain or cyanosis of the lips should be examined accordingly. Arterial blood gases should be checked together with computed tomography of the thorax and/or ventilation-perfusion scintigraphy if needed. These symptoms can also develop due to excessive resection and closure under tension without any demonstrable thromboembolic event especially in patients with centripedal obesity.

10.7 Conclusions

Abdominoplasty is shaping of the abdomen and surrounding areas considering the trunk as an aesthetic unit. Like any surgical procedure, it has its own drawbacks and complications, and the possibilities should be discussed with patient before the operation. If a patient is informed in detail before abdominoplasty, most of the arguable problems will be prevented after the operation. The end result of abdominoplasty is equally dependent on the body habitus of the patient and technical aspects of the operation. Patient selection is extremely important, and patients who are candidates of potential complications are not so hard to foresee. Patients with a BMI greater than or equal to 30 have a greater complication rate. Surgical technique should be individualized according to the needs of the patient's body habitus. If the degree of deformity does not seem to be suitable for a single-stage correction, surgeon should certainly inform the patient and plan two or three stages of correction. Degree of delamination and amount of liposuction should be optimal in order to avoid perfusion problems which lead to collateral problems. Postoperative care is detailed compared to many of the other aesthetic operations. Early mobilization, incremental increase in daily activities, and control of diet will ensure minimization of complications. The surgeon should know that patients undergoing abdominoplasty and concomitant procedures have considerable risk of readmission to hospital even after a month of the surgery [19].

References

1. Winocour J, Gupta V, Ramirez JR, Shack RB, Grotting JC, Higdon KK. Abdominoplasty: risk factors, complication rates, and safety of combined procedures. Plast Reconstr Surg. 2015;136(5):597e–606. doi:10.1097/PRS.0000000000001700.
2. Amato MC, Pizzolanti G, Torregrossa V, Misiano G, Milano S, Giordano C. Visceral adiposity index (VAI) is predictive of an altered adipokine profile in patients with type 2 diabetes. PLoS One. 2014;9(3):e91969. doi:10.1371/journal.pone.0091969. eCollection 2014.
3. Suder A, Plonka M, Jagielski P, Piorecka B, Glodzik J. Physiological and environmental factors associated with central fat distribution in pubertal girls. J Physiol Pharmacol. 2015;66(3):463–70.
4. Cardwell SM, Crandon JL, Nicolau DP, McClure MH, Nailor MD. Epidemiology and economics of adult patients hospitalized with urinary tract infections. Hosp Pract (1995). 2016;44(1):1–8.

5. Campbell W, Pierson J, Cohen-Shohet R, Mast BA. Maximizing chemoprophylaxis against venous thromboembolism in abdominoplasty patients with the use of preoperative heparin administration. Ann Plast Surg. 2014;72(6):S94–6. doi:10.1097/SAP.0000000000000132.
6. Rogliani M, Silvi E, Labardi L, Maggiulli F, Cervelli V. Obese and nonobese patients: complications of abdominoplasty. Ann Plast Surg. 2006;57(3):336–8.
7. Rieger UM, Erba P, Wettstein R, Schumacher R, Schwenzer-Zimmerer K, Haug M, Pierer G, Kalbermatten DF. Does abdominoplasty with liposuction of the love handles yield a shorter scar? An analysis with abdominal 3D laser scanning. Ann Plast Surg. 2008;61(4):359–63. doi:10.1097/SAP.0b013e31816d824a.
8. Keaney TC, Tanzi E, Alster T. Comparison of 532 nm Potassium Titanyl Phosphate Laser and 595 nm pulsed dye laser in the treatment of erythematous surgical scars: a randomized, controlled, open-label study. Dermatol Surg. 2016;42(1):70–6. doi:10.1097/DSS.0000000000000582.
9. Swanson E. Comparison of limited and full dissection abdominoplasty using laser fluorescence imaging to evaluate perfusion of the abdominal skin. Plast Reconstr Surg. 2015;136(1):31e–43. doi:10.1097/PRS.0000000000001376.
10. Shestak KC. The extended abdominoplasty. Clin Plast Surg. 2014;41(4):705–13. doi:10.1016/j.cps.2014.07.001.
11. Swanson E. Prospective clinical study of 551 cases of liposuction and abdominoplasty performed individually and in combination. Plast Reconstr Surg Glob Open. 2013;1(5):e32. doi:10.1097/GOX.0b013e3182a333d7. eCollection 2013.
12. Valença-Filipe R, Martins A, Silva Á, Vásconez LO, Amarante J, Costa-Ferreira A. Dissection technique for abdominoplasty: a prospective study on scalpel versus diathermocoagulation (coagulation mode). Plast Reconstr Surg Glob Open. 2015;3(1):e299. doi:10.1097/GOX.0000000000000222. eCollection 2015.
13. Marsh DJ, Fox A, Grobbelaar AO, Chana JS. Abdominoplasty and seroma: a prospective randomised study comparing scalpel and handheld electrocautery dissection. J Plast Reconstr Aesthet Surg. 2015;68(2):192–6. doi:10.1016/j.bjps.2014.10.004. Epub 2014 Oct 13.
14. Epstein S, Epstein MA, Gutowski KA. Lipoabdominoplasty without drains or progressive tension sutures: an analysis of 100 consecutive patients. Aesthet Surg J. 2015;35(4):434–40. doi:10.1093/asj/sju049.
15. Quaba AA, Conlin S, Quaba O. The no-drain, no-quilt abdominoplasty: a single-surgeon series of 271 patients. Plast Reconstr Surg. 2015;135(3):751–60. doi:10.1097/PRS.0000000000001031.
16. Friedman T, Coon D, Kanbour-Shakir A, Michaels J, Rubin JP. Defining the lymphatic system of the anterior abdominal wall: an anatomical study. Plast Reconstr Surg. 2015;135(4):1027–32. doi:10.1097/PRS.0000000000001136.
17. Horch RE. Incisional negative pressure wound therapy for high-risk wounds. J Wound Care. 2015;24(4 Suppl):21–8. doi:10.12968/jowc.2015.24.Sup4b.21.
18. Seruya M, Venturi ML, lorio ML, Davison SP. Efficacy and safety of venous thromboembolism prophylaxis in highest risk plastic surgery patients. Plast Reconstr Surg. 2008;122:1702–8.
19. Massenburg BB, Sanati-Mehrizy P, Jablonka EM, Taub PJ. Risk factors for readmission and adverse outcomes in abdominoplasty. Plast Reconstr Surg. 2015;136(5):968–77. doi:10.1097/PRS.0000000000001680.

Chapter 11
Postoperative Care

Esin Aksungur

Postoperative care is as important as the surgery itself in terms of the success of the operation and prevention of complications. No matter how successful the operation is, if you cannot ensure the postoperative comfort of the patient and cannot manage the postoperative period well, this success will be shadowed.

The smallest detail omitted in the postoperative period may trigger other problems and lead to undesirable problems.

The planning of postoperative period begins with the first consultation with the patient. Information such as the general health status of the patient and the presence, if any, of additional diseases is essential for postoperative care. The operational area, size of operation, and procedures applied in the operation are other significant parameters defining the postoperative process [1].

The most important criteria defining the postoperative period in abdominoplasty are:

1. Additional health problems
2. Age and weight
3. Anesthesia time
4. Amount of excised tissue
5. Amount of fat removed through liposuction
6. Amount of plication on the rectus fascia

Postoperative care starts with the dressing of the surgical area and ends when the patient goes back to fully functional normal life. After being discharged from the operative room, patients spend the first 24–48 h in the hospital. In this period, many factors affect the prognosis of the postoperative period. Most important are pain control, blood pressure and drain follow-up, and prevention of early complications like deep vein thrombosis (DVT) and thromboembolism (TE) and hematoma.

E. Aksungur
Department of Plastic Surgery, Florence Nightingale Hospital, Istanbul, Turkey
e-mail: eaksungur@gmail.com

K.T. Tiryaki (ed.), *Inverse Abdominoplasty*, DOI 10.1007/978-3-319-39310-0_11

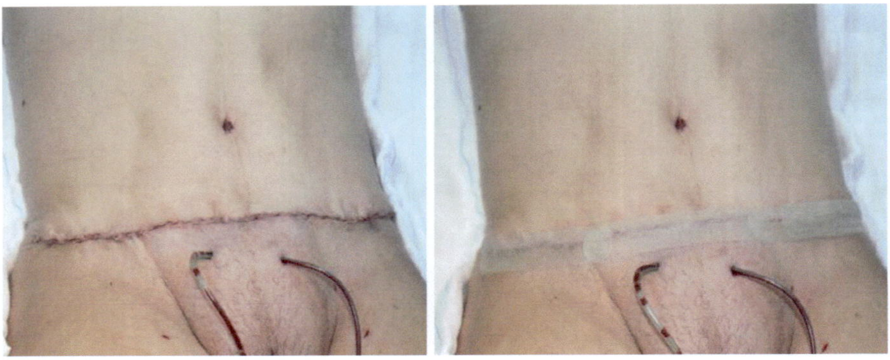

Picture 11.1 Covering the incision line with strips

11.1 Postoperative Dressings

In order to reduce postoperative edema and ensure hemostasis, pressure dressings are applied. The first step is to cover the incision line. Different dressing techniques can be used to cover the incision line. Antibiotic pomades, sterile gauze dressing, or strips directly covering the incision line can be used.

We prefer covering the suture line with elastic strips for 2 weeks. Changing the strips at the end of the first week, covering them again after cleaning the incision line, and keeping them covered for one more week protect the incision line for a long time and eliminate the need for wound care. After 72 h of the normal epithelialization period, the patients are allowed to take a shower with these waterproof strips (Picture 11.1).

The umbilical area requires special attention. Protecting the suture line in this area from maceration is highly important. The dressing applied to this area with antibiotic pomades during the operation is uncovered on the third day at the first dressing change, and it can be left uncovered since epithelialization is completed then. It is enough to clean and put pomade on the area daily over 10 days. One should be careful in cases of redness and discharge in this area and try to control the local infection in the early period with oral antibiotics and sterilizing agents used for wound care, if necessary (Picture 11.2).

Desired abdominal shape is ensured in the early period by pressure applied on the nature-identical sulci created on the midline and as lateral to the rectus. Besides, with pressure on these areas, the flaps adhere to the base within a short time and the risk of complications, such as seroma, decreases [2]. After the gauze sponges are placed, the abdomen is pressured with tensile bands from the lower end of the costa to the suprapubic area (Pictures 11.3, 11.4). The corset worn over all these dressing should be used for 3 weeks (Picture 11.5).

This dressing can be removed after the postoperative third day or can be maintained up to 1 week depending on the surgeon's choice. Dressings, apart from strips, do not need to be replaced after removal. After checking the suture line and umbilical area and explaining the daily abdominal care to the patient, a corset can be worn.

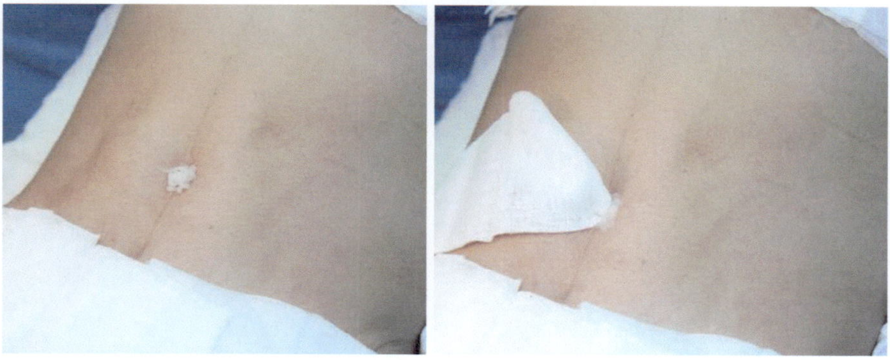

Picture 11.2 Umbilical area dressing

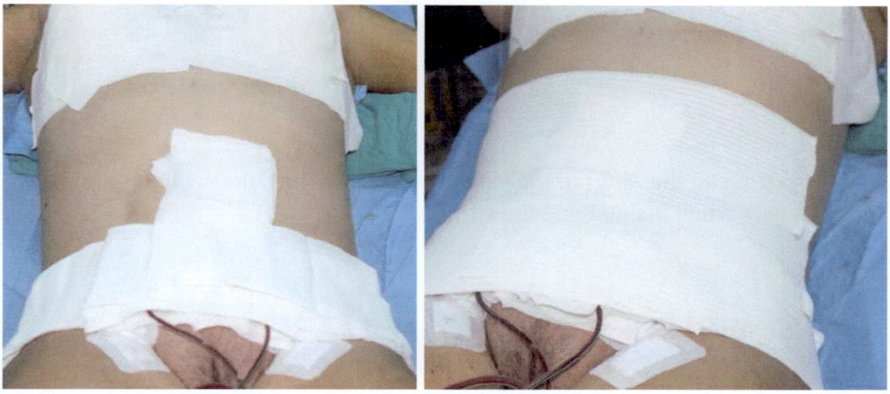

Picture 11.3 Abdominal dressing after covering the incision line after operation. Placing the sponges and covering with tensile plasters

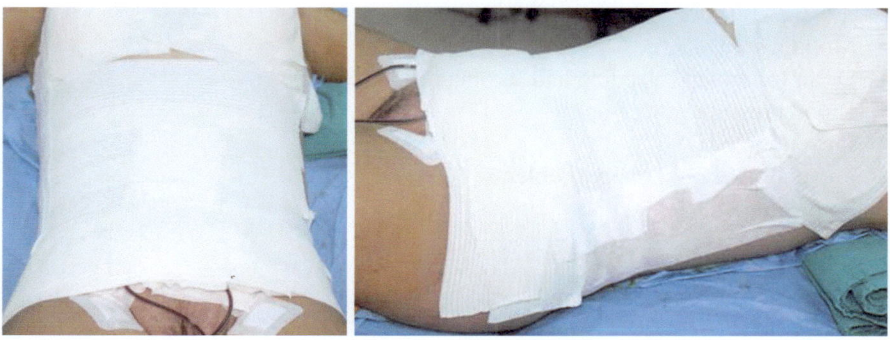

Picture 11.4 Covering the whole abdominal area with tensile plasters

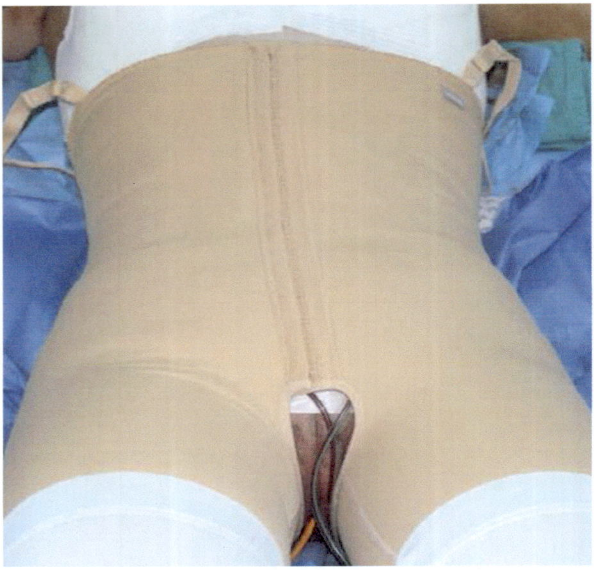

Picture 11.5 View of patient with corset worn over the dressing

After removing all dressings of the patient on the third day, the patient is allowed to take a shower while maintaining the strips.

11.2 Hospital Follow-Up

Postoperative hospital care varies for every patient. It typically falls between 24 and 72 h. If all goes well in the follow-up of the patient, the patient can be discharged from the hospital within 24 h.

The parameters to be followed are:

- Mobilization
- Drain follow-up (bleeding and seroma follow-up)
- Blood pressure follow-up
- Prevention of DVT
- Prevention of pulmonary problems
- Pain control

11.2.1 Mobilization

The patients are encouraged to get mobilized as soon as the sixth hour postoperatively. This is important for the prevention of many complications like respiratory insufficiency and DVT.

11.2.2 Drain Follow-Up

Prevention of early hematoma is of primary importance in the postoperative period. Rates of hematoma reported in the literature are in the range of 0.8–3 % [3].

Another problem, which is observed more frequently than hematoma, is seroma in abdominoplasty follow-up [4]. It arises when lymphatics in the deep fat tissue are damaged after surgery. While bleeding is observed frequently within the first 24 h, the incidence of seroma increases later on. Therefore, there are various protocols for follow-up of patients with drains. There are protocols recommending follow-up up to 7 days with drains to avoid from seroma in patients with wide dissections. In addition, other protective methods tried include decreasing dead space with sutures or facilitating adherence of the flap to the base with fibrin glue and protecting the Scarpa fascia on the base during the dissection [5].

However, since there is no wide dissection in our technique with minimal dead space, we use only closed drain systems. We keep drains until less than 30–40 cc/24 h and their contents become serous. This process is usually completed within the first 24 h in many patients. Depending on the surgeon's choice, two silicon or Jackson-Pratt drains placed on the incision line or suprapubic area will be enough.

Postoperative hematoma or seroma generally restrict themselves; however, if the accumulated blood is not detected in the early period, it may lead to necrosis on the flap area due to the pressure it causes and wound healing problems due to tightness on the suture line [6]. In suspicious cases, the abdomen should be checked by removing the dressing. Ultrasonography (USG) is the most valuable method in early period diagnosis. While it is difficult to discharge hematoma with an injector in the early period, it becomes easier due to fall of fibrin within the following days.

11.2.3 Blood Pressure Follow-Up

While a TA follow-up with 4–6-h intervals within the first 24 h after operation is enough for patients with no hypertension problems, this must be more frequent for patients with previous medical history. Preoperatively used medication must be screened carefully, and any existing antihypertensive drugs must be continued. Severe pain and improper liquid uptake in the postoperative period may lead to fluctuations in tension values of patients. Hypertension problems in the early period are the most important risk factors increasing the hematoma [7].

One should be careful with the liquid treatment and avoid charging excessive volumes to the patient. Cardiology consultation should be requested for patients who still have tension fluctuations and TA values over 150–100 mmHg despite meeting all these criteria [8].

11.2.4 Prevention of Deep Vein Thrombosis

Venous thrombosis begins in areas in stasis, particularly on the small veins in the legs. Hypercoagulability associated with surgical stress and trauma increases the risk of venous thrombosis associated with hypotonia on the leg muscles during anesthesia. Thrombosis is firstly caused by the obstruction in the vein [9]. If the obstructed vein is a major vein, distal venous pressure increases and edema occurs in the extremity. Rupture of the clot may occur and its embolization of the right heart and then the lungs threatens life [10].

Early postoperative mobilization is highly important to reduce venous stasis and prevent venous thromboembolism. Thromboembolic deterrent stocking and intra- and postoperative intermittent pneumatic compression boots worn during the operation and maintained within the first 24 h are the most important protection methods against thromboembolism [11, 12]. Low-molecular-weight heparin (LMWH) shall be the routine treatment in patients with major tissue removal and high-volume liposuction. SC Fraxiparine can be applied 1 h before the surgery. The doses up to 40 mg/g would not increase the risk of bleeding and can be used with confidence [13].

In healthy patients who do not have additional problems and achieve early postoperative mobilization, the abovementioned measures are enough. However, for patients with risk factors, a more detailed examination must be performed, and appropriate treatment shall be planned.

In 2011, the American Society of Plastic Surgeons' task force compiled recommendations for thromboembolism prophylaxis in patients undergoing plastic surgery procedures including body contouring. Risk factors are defined in accordance with the 2005 Caprini Risk Assessment Model (RAM), and the risk group and treatment protocol to be applied to the patient were determined [14] (Tables 11.1 and 11.2).

11.2.5 Prevention of Pulmonary Problems

Early mobilization and good respiratory physiotherapy are essential for protecting patients from many postoperative complications. Intra-abdominal pressure is increased due to plication applied to the front wall of the abdomen during operation. This means confining the lungs to a more narrow area, thereby decreasing the pulmonary capacity. In this way, the pulmonary base is inactivated, particularly in patients whose respiration is superficialized due to postoperative pain and who cannot respire actively. Superficial coughing cannot discharge the secretion occurring in the lungs, and therefore, mucus obturators may trigger atelectasis by blocking the basal alveoli in the lung [15].

Table 11.1 Risk factors for venous thromboembolism based on the 2005 caprini risk assessment model

One point for each risk factor	Two points for each risk factor	Three points for each risk factor
Age 41–60 years	Age 60–74 years	Age over 75 years
Minor surgery planned	Malignancy (previous or present)	History of DVT/PE
History of prior major surgery (<1 month)	Major surgery (>45 min)	Family history of thrombosis
Varicose veins	Patient confined to bed (>72 h)	Positive factor V Leiden
History of inflammatory bowel disease	Central venous access	Positive prothrombin 20210A
Swollen legs (current)		Elevated serum homocysteine
Obesity		Positive lupus anticoagulant
Sepsis (<1 month)		Elevated anticardiolipin antibodies
Serious lung disease (>1 month)		Heparin-induced thrombocytopenia
Abnormal pulmonary function (COPD)		Other congenital or acquired thrombophilia
Other risk factors		
For women only		
Oral contraceptives or hormone replacement therapy		
Pregnancy or postpartum (<1 month)		
History of unexplained stillborn infant Recurrent spontaneous abortion, premature Birth with toxemia or growth-restricted infant		

Table 11.2 Measures to prevent venous thromboembolism in patients undergoing body contouring performed under general anesthesia lasting more than 60 min

2005 caprini RAM score	Recommendations
3–6	Should consider the option to use postoperative LMWH or unfractionated heparin
3 or more	Should consider the option to utilize mechanical prophylaxis throughout the duration of chemical prophylaxis for nonambulatory patients
7 or more	Should strongly consider the option to use extended LMWH postoperative prophylaxis (up to 4 weeks)

The stasis in pulmonary base may lead to atelectasis and more severe pulmonary problems, in particular:

- In patients with pulmonary problems before operation
- In patients on whom excessive plication is applied during operation
- In patients with intra-abdominal fat

Respiratory exercises must be started in the early period.

The oxygen saturation of the patients is followed up, and patients with less than 95 % oxygen saturation in normal room pressure should be supported with nasal O_2. Bronchodilator treatment must absolutely be embedded for the patients with rales in respiration sounds, and respiratory physiotherapy must be continued during this treatment [16].

11.2.6 Pain Control

Pain is one of the most significant problems in postoperative period in abdominoplasty. Pain might be the underlying cause for many problems, and it can be prevented with good postoperative analgesia.

Sensorial, effective, motivational, and cognitive components of pain are closely associated with the pain perceptions, senses, and experiences of a person. In fact, the pain perception of a person can be managed with simple methods [17]. The first phase of this method must be to reduce stress. Information provided before operation, a patient's recognition of what they will face, and their trust in the team and surgeon reduce the stress factor. Studies have demonstrated that decreasing preoperative general anxiety level reduces PCA need. It has been found that there is a positive correlation between preoperative sudden anxiety and postoperative pain and hospitalization time [18].

Perioperative local anesthesia or blocks facilitate a powerful pain control in the postoperative period. Abdominal fascia is an area with high pain tenderness, and plication in this area is the primary reason for postoperative pain in abdominoplasty. A long-lasting effective pain control can be achieved with local anesthetic injections under the fascia, which is described in detail in the surgical technique chapter.

The importance of pain treatment are as follows:

- It reduces pulmonary problems. A patient with less pain can inspire deeply and respiration is not superficialized. Activating pulmonary basal with deep inspiration and reducing secretion through coughing minimize postoperative pulmonary problems.

Table 11.3 The risk of complications increases due to the lack of pain control

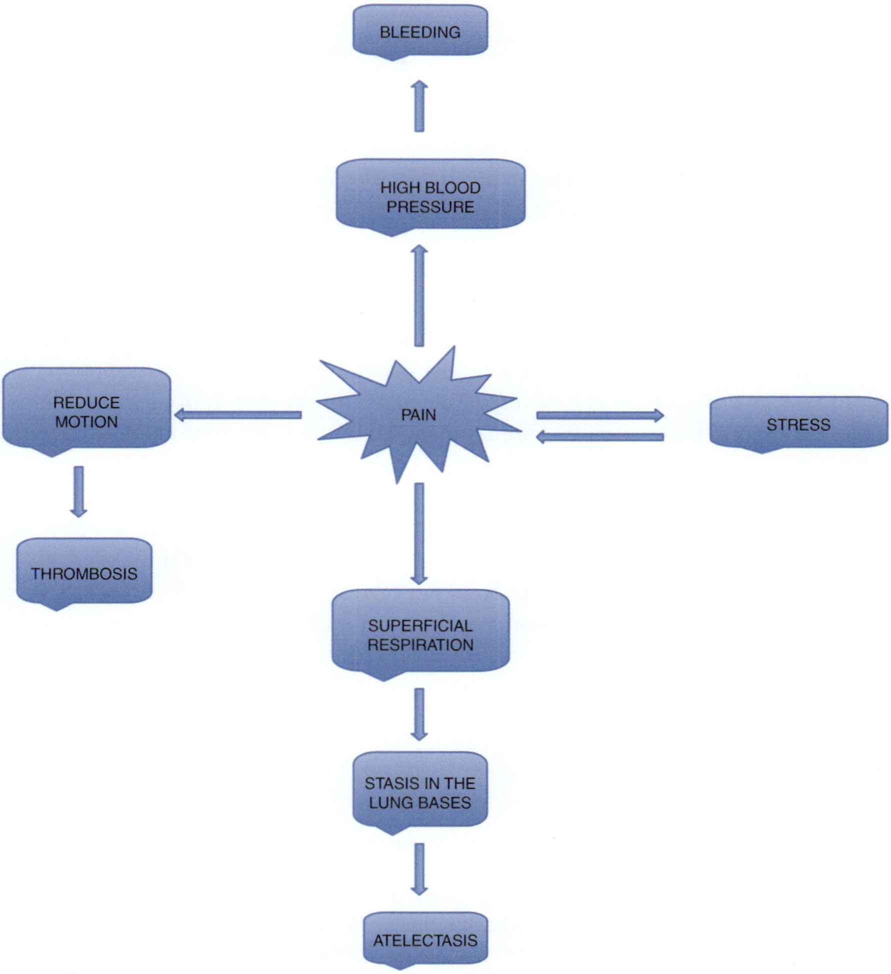

- Excessive pain activates sympathetic system and may lead to blood pressure instabilities. This may increase the risk of hematoma.
- It leads to agitation of patient. High anxiety increases the tenderness of person against pain and leads to exaggeration of pain perception. The first few postoperative hours are very important for pain perception. Pain is defined as a physiological-psychological experience. In the studies performed, if the patient feels excessive pain in the early period, his pain perception changes, and he feels pain longer and more severely. In patients without early postoperative pain, pain tolerance in the late period is much higher.
- Early mobilization is highly difficult in patients with pain, which is the golden standard in prevention of thromboembolic incidences (Table 11.3).

11.3 House Follow-Up

The use of antibiotics and anti-inflammatory medication for 5 days is a routine. Patients with pulmonary diseases must continue their respiratory exercises for 1 week.

Fever and fatigue beginning after the third day shall raise suspicion of a surgical infection, and in this case, appropriate diagnostic tests are mandatory. In patient groups with emboli risks, heparin prophylaxis can be continued in accordance with the patient's score.

In addition to all these treatments, some of the most frequent problems discomfiting the patient in the postoperative period are gastrointestinal problems. Particularly in patients with excessive plication, problems such as reduction in intestinal movements and constipation may occur. Profuse liquid consumption and motility-regulating drugs can be recommended for patients with such problems. These complaints are usually temporary and intestinal activity turns to normal within 10–15 days.

The first visit is usually on the third day, with the removal of the heavy bandage, and the patient can take a shower with suture lines covered with strips. They can usually continue their basic daily routines after the postoperative third day.

The patients can go back to work at the end of the first week; however, they should be asked to avoid exercise increasing intra-abdominal pressure for 3 months after surgery.

References

1. Klein JA. Post-tumescent liposuction care: open drainage and bimodal compression. Dermatol Clin. 1999;17(4):881–9.
2. Grazer F. Expert commentary. Plast Surg. 1989;2:44–50.
3. Araco A, Sorge R, Overton J, Araco F, Gravante G. Postbariatric patients undergoing body-contouring abdominoplasty: two techniques to raise the flap and their influence on postoperative complications. Ann Plast Surg. 2009;62(6):613–7.
4. Matarasso A, Matarasso DM, Matarasso EJ. Abdominoplasty: classic principles and technique. Clin Plast Surg. 2014;41(4):655–72.
5. Bercial ME, Sabino Neto M, Calil JA, Rossetto LA, Ferreira LM. Suction drains, quilting sutures, and fibrin sealant in the prevention of seroma formation in abdominoplasty: which is the best strategy? Aesthetic Plast Surg. 2012;36(2):370–3. doi:10.1007/s00266-011-9807-8. Epub 2011 Aug 20.
6. Pollock H, Pollock T. Progressive tension sutures: a technique to reduce local complications in abdominoplasty. Plast Reconstr Surg. 2000;105:2583–6.
7. Estafanous FG. Hypertension in the surgical patient: management of blood pressure and anesthesia. Cleve Clin J Med. 1989;56(4):385–93.
8. Thompson D, Ampel L. Perioperative hypertension. The primary care physician's role. Postgrad Med. 1988;84(2):261–3, 266–8.
9. Reish RG, Damjanocic B, Colwell AS. Deep venous thrombosis prophylaxis in body contouring:105 consecutive patients. Ann Plast Surg. 2012;69(4):412–4.

10. Storti S, Crucitti P, Cina G. Risk factors and prevention of venous thromboembolism. Rays. 1996;21:439–60.
11. Tapson VF, Shirvanian S. Venous thromboembolism: identifying patients at risk and establishing prophylaxis. Curr Med Res Opin. 2015;28:1–64.
12. Conroy FJ, Thornton DJ, Mather DP, Srinvasan J, Hart NB. Thromboembolic prophylaxis in plastic surgery: a 12-year follow-up in the UK. J Plast Reconstr Aesthet Surg. 2006;59(5):510–4.
13. Newall G, Ruiz-Razura A, Mentz HA, Patronella CK, Ibarra FR, Zarak A. A retrospective study on the use of low-molecular-weight heparin for thromboembolism prophylaxis in large volume liposuction and body contouring procedures. Aesthetic Plast Surg. 2006;30(1):86–95.
14. Murphy Jr RX, Alderman A, Gutowski K, Kerrigan C, Rosolowski K, Schechter L, Schmitz D, Wilkins E. Evidence-based practices for thromboembolism references prevention: summary of the ASPS venous thromboembolism task force report. Plast Reconstr Surg. 2012;130(1):168e–75.
15. Jansen DA, Kaye AD, Banister RE, Madan AK, Hyde KG, Nossaman BD. Changes in compliance predict pulmonary morbidity in patients undergoing abdominal plication. Plast Reconstr Surg. 1999;103(7):2012–5.
16. Rodrigues MA, Nahas FX, Gomes HC, Ferreira LM. Ventilatory function and intra-abdominal pressure in patients who underwent abdominoplasty with plication of the external oblique aponeurosis. Aesthetic Plast Surg. 2013;37(5):993–9. doi:10.1007/s00266-013-0158-5. Epub 2013 Aug 27.
17. Tang J, Gibson SJ. Psychological evaluation of relationship between trait anxiety, pain perception and reduced state anxiety. J Pain. 2005;6(9):12–9.
18. Sjoling M, Nordahal G, Olofsson N. The impact of preoperative information on state anxiety, postoperative pain and satisfaction with pain management. Patient Educ Couns. 2003;51:169–76.

MIX
Papier aus verantwortungsvollen Quellen
Paper from responsible sources
FSC® C105338
FSC
www.fsc.org

If you have any concerns about our products,
you can contact us on
ProductSafety@springernature.com

In case Publisher is established outside the EU,
the EU authorized representative is:
Springer Nature Customer Service Center GmbH
Europaplatz 3, 69115 Heidelberg, Germany

Printed by Libri Plureos GmbH
in Hamburg, Germany